Wisdom from a Chair:

Thirty Years of Quadriplegia

Published by BookLocker.com, Inc., Bradenton, Florida, U.S.A.

Printed on acid-free paper.

BookLocker.com, Inc.
2016

First Edition

Cover art: Don Quixote mounted on a wheelchair and fighting the windmills of injustice. Artist: Mitchell Batavia

Wisdom from a Chair:

Thirty Years of Quadriplegia

The Memoirs of Andrew I. Batavia

Andrew I. Batavia
Mitchell Batavia

Dedicated to my wonderful children,
Joe and Katey Batavia,
who have contributed enormously to the joy in my life,
and who will, hopefully, learn the lessons of my disability,
which should contribute to the joy in theirs.

A.I.B.

Table of Contents

Forewords

During the twenty-fifth anniversary year of the Americans with Disabilities Act, it is only fitting that the recently discovered memoirs of Andrew Batavia be published to share the amazing life journey of a man who at the age of sixteen broke his neck, sustaining a high-level spinal cord injury, and nevertheless overcame huge obstacles to have a spectacular career fighting for the civil rights of those with disabilities.

Instead of dwelling on self-pity and dependency, Drew responded to his challenge, attending Harvard Law School and Stanford Medical School's public health program, serving as a White House Fellow, achieving tenure at Florida International University at the full professor rank, and leading the fight as a civil rights disability activist.

As a White House Fellow in 1990, Drew worked as a special assistant to me at the Department of Justice while I served as attorney general of the United States. In that role, he helped draft the language and write the regulations needed to implement the Americans with Disabilities Act, a landmark civil rights act for the disability community. People with disabilities would no longer be treated as second-class citizens.

Drew served as a role model for productivity, despite having no use of his hands or legs. He published more than 120 journal articles, books, book chapters, letters to the editor, newspaper articles, and book reviews during his brief lifetime. And he accomplished this with only a few inexpensive work accommodations: a computer, a reading stand, a mouth stick, and a raised desk area. Despite all this productivity, he still had time to serve his government, contribute to his community, and raise a family.

Drew's vision, energy, and high standards symbolized the spirit captured in a knockoff Picasso print that hung on his office wall. In the print, Don Quixote charges a windmill. But instead of sitting on his horse, he is mounted on a wheelchair. In a similar manner, Drew spent his life charging the windmills of injustice in order to right wrongs.

Drew showed us what can be accomplished despite severe disability. We can all learn from the wisdom he acquired during his lifetime.

Dick Thornburgh
Former Attorney General of the United States and
Governor of Pennsylvania

My friend, Drew Batavia, was an intelligent, industrious, accomplished individual who crammed an impressive amount of purposeful living into his too-short life. A quick review of his resume confirms the observation.

President of his high school class, graduate with honors from UC Riverside, JD from Harvard Law School, master's from Stanford. He was a White House Fellow during George H. W. Bush's presidency; associate director of the White House Domestic Policy Council; and special assistant to the attorney general of the United States. He served as the executive director of the National Council on Disability. I got to know him when he was writing regulations for the Americans with Disabilities Act, which I had cosponsored and strongly supported. Not long after, I asked him to work in my office as our legislative assistant on health care issues. He agreed and worked for me for a couple years. Lucky me. After he left our office, he practiced law as a partner in a Miami law firm and taught public health policy at Florida International University. After their move to Miami, he and his wonderful wife, Cheryl, adopted two children from a Siberian orphanage, Joe and Katerina, who made their busy lives all the busier and fulfilled. Drew died from an infection in 2003 at the age of forty-five. He had managed to do many important things in his too-few years. People blessed with twice his lifespan would be proud to have lived so accomplished a life. And he would have done a great deal more had he not died so young.

That brief, crammed paragraph should convince the reader that Drew Batavia was a person of enormous ability. And that is exactly who he was, a man of great ability. If you were lucky enough to know him personally, as I was, you knew also that he was a man with passion, warmth, kindness, joyfulness, and a confident determination to make every day of his life matter to himself and to others. And you would know he was a person with quadriplegia using a motorized wheelchair, which he controlled by moving his chin, since his sixteenth year, when he was grievously injured in an automobile accident.

Drew deserves to be remembered for what he did, not for what happened to him. He earned that respect. Of course, he's all the more impressive for having lived such a successful life while facing in every hour of every day such an imposing adversity. But he was first and foremost a capable, reliable, smart, opinionated, determined, and useful human being, a guy you could count on and look up to.

I'm one of many people who had the good fortune to be inspired by Drew's character and example. I'm a better man for having known him, and I'll never forget him. Now, people who weren't privileged to have known Drew when he was with us can get to know him in this memoir, discovered only recently by his family and completed by Drew's brother, Mitchell. In these pages you hear Drew's voice tell Drew's story: how a man of great ability put his whole heart and soul and all his many talents into making our country a better place for all of us. It's the story of a hero.

John McCain
United States Senator

Preface

I believe the key to happiness is to find a good mission in life, to make it your life's work, to take that work very seriously, and not to take yourself seriously at all. Most people who publish autobiographies are self-important, self-serving blowhards, who take themselves much too seriously. With some notable exceptions, this is true whether the author is a sports hero, captain of industry, or even president of the United States. Publishing one's private memoirs is, in a sense, the ultimate act of arrogance, in that it assumes that someone else would, or even should, be interested in the author's existence.

So, this raises the obvious question: Why did I write and publish this particular memoir, particularly at the relatively young age of forty-five, without being famous yet, or possibly ever. One possible answer, of course, is that I am a self-important, self-serving blowhard. I cannot be objective about this, so I will leave it to you to make this judgment by the end of the book. Another possibility, however, is that a depiction of my life and my mission can make some unique contribution to our understanding of the world. I like to think that this is the case; yet, again, one's ability to assess the uniqueness of one's own life objectively while in the process of living it is limited. In fact, everyone's life is to some extent unique, and some of the most interesting and insightful life stories are those of the so-called "average citizen" rather than the rich and famous. I recognize that this is sacrilege in our celebrity-oriented society, in which those of us who are not on some Social Register A-list, and therefore have not risen to the public consciousness, do not exist, for all practical purposes.

However, there are reasons that my life may offer unique insights. First, for the last thirty years, I have not gone to a single public place or event in which I have not been part of the show. People appear infinitely interested in watching me racing down the street in my chin-controlled, motorized wheelchair. Often I would be accompanied by one or both of my beautiful children, whom my wife and I adopted from Russia; one would be standing on the back of the chair and the other sitting on my foot plates, and we would be weaving in and out among people at full speed.

Living one's life without the use of arms, legs, or hands presents some interesting challenges and appears to be inherently intriguing to many people. I suppose some are wondering what my life is like and whether they could survive under similar circumstances; I am sure that most could, in that we humans have a remarkable capacity to adapt to almost any conditions. I have never resented this voyeurism; as a person who was not disabled for the first sixteen years of my life, I am certain that I would have been similarly curious if I had not severed my spinal cord in 1973 and if I were in the same room as someone with my current disability.

Yet this still does not quite answer the question as to why my life warrants the sacrifice of trees necessary to publish this book. Although my disability—high-level quadriplegia—is relatively rare and was even more so thirty years ago, there have always been a fair number of people with quadriplegia who had survived back in the 1950s, and there are other disabilities that are far more rare and debilitating than mine. However, there have been very few people with my level of disability who have studied in, worked in, lived in, or even visited the places I have been, such as Harvard Law School, Stanford Medical School, the US Attorney General's Office, the White House, the Senate, and the top of the Great Wall of China.

These particular experiences do not make my life more important than those of my colleagues with disabilities who have not experienced these places. I remember, when I was in rehabilitation at the famous Rusk Institute in New York, that virtually every one of my fellow inmates with a recently acquired disability had a story that was sufficiently interesting for a book or a motion picture. In fact, years later I watched the movie *The Waterdance*, which brilliantly told the story of a person with quadriplegia adapting to his disability. Much to my satisfaction, it was told in a refreshingly honest manner, warts and all. Although this film was based on a particular individual, it describes well the general experience of many of us becoming rehabilitated. I recommend it strongly.

One of the reasons that such stories are so interesting is that they deal with a very intense situation—going through the transition from being a "normal, able-bodied" person to a "cripple," "invalid," "gimp," "handicapped person," or "person with a disability," depending upon how you are addressed, where you live, and with whom you interact. My experiences have been particularly intense, in that they have taken place in some of the most competitive and respected institutions of our society. I believe that such intense experiences often offer great insight for those who survive them, much as Viktor Frankl derived remarkable insights from his horrible personal experiences as a survivor of the Holocaust and John McCain gained a unique perspective from his five and a half years as a POW in Vietnam. This is not to compare their horrendous experiences with the experiences of quadriplegia (although the permanence of quadriplegia does provide some similar intensity); the purpose is only to indicate that all such experiences offer the promise of wisdom to those willing to learn their lessons.

The title of this book may require some explanation. Generally speaking, very limited wisdom can be derived from inanimate objects, such as chairs. A notable exception is the wisdom that can be gained from a wheelchair. Wheelchairs are among the most vilified objects in human history. Even as we enter the new millennium, it is common to turn on the local news and hear some commentator talking about a person who is "wheelchair-bound," "confined to a wheelchair," or even "condemned to a wheelchair." Those of us who use motorized wheelchairs do not find them confining, binding, or condemning; they expand our horizons and help us get where we want to go, often more expediently and faster than the legs of our colleagues.

Wheelchairs have been used in virtually every medium, including novels and films, to depict weakness, evil, and other negative traits. Their use in horror films, such as *Psycho,* is practically ubiquitous. In the final, ironic scene of the movie *Sleeper,* Woody Allen portrays the leader of the world as being a person in a wheelchair, apparently suggesting that such a thing would be impossible (despite the fact that FDR led us out of the Depression and to victory in World War II from his wheelchair). This particular negative portrayal does not offend me as much as it amuses me. A wheelchair and life in a wheelchair are not negative things in themselves. A wheelchair is actually almost always a positive thing, as long as it is functional and affordable, and the life of a person with a disability can be very good or very bad, depending in part on the individual's circumstances and what he or she is able to do with them. Although disability is often associated with adversity, it can also be a source of very positive things, such as wisdom, for those who are open to it.

Over the years, many people have told me that I am an inspiration. Although I have always appreciated such sentiments when conveyed sincerely and without pity, for a long time I found such compliments somewhat annoying. I always find "inspirational movies" about the lives of people with disabilities a little nauseating. My mission in this world is to try to ensure that all people, including people with disabilities, have greater choices in and control over their lives. I believe that achieving this mission will make the world a slightly better place than it was before I got here. Recently, I have decided that if this orientation, or the way in which I live my life, inspires someone, that is fine.

I imagine that there are some who do not share my view of a better world and who think what I do makes it a little worse, and there are some who will no doubt be offended by some of the things I say in this book. Although such offense is not intended, it is also fine. I pride myself as one of the early opponents of the notion of "political correctness," even before political incorrectness was fashionable, and I believe first and foremost in honesty expressed in a sensitive manner, even when it does not please everyone. I take what I have characterized as a "constructively cynical" approach to life, and I leave few of our cherished institutions unexamined.

Finally, after hopefully having at least partially justified this book, I must answer the question as to why I am writing it now. On August 12, 2003, I will celebrate the thirtieth anniversary of my spinal cord injury. Every year, I celebrate another year of survival with my disability, and it seems that a thirtieth anniversary should be commemorated in a special way.

I have written this book primarily as a gift to my children, Joe and Katey, to whom it is dedicated. In writing it, I estimate that my audience will be somewhere between fifty close friends, relatives, and colleagues and a couple of million people who I know less well. This is a substantially larger variation than the readership of my two previous academic books, which sold a few thousand copies. I will be happy either way, though I will be particularly gratified if this very personal book reaches a large audience.

Several years ago, one of my close relatives indicated that she wanted to write a biography about me, apparently more impressed with my achievements than I was at the time. I told her that I would be ready to have my life story in print once I had achieved something of note. I did not tell her, but I was also concerned that, because she is too close to me emotionally, she would not be able to maintain objectivity and the piece would inevitably have been one of those inspirational things that make me sick. I needed someone much more critical of me to write such a book, such as me.

I am not certain whether my other criterion has been met, and the reader will have to judge whether I have achieved anything of note at this stage of my life. Irrespective of the satisfaction of this criterion, I am writing this now in part because one of the key insights I have derived from my disability is not to take anything for granted. Although I am very healthy generally, and few "able-bodied people" could keep up with me throughout my long workday, I have had several severe acute episodes over the years in which I came close to dying. Such occasional near-death experiences are part of the territory associated with quadriplegia. One of the reasons I am writing this book now is in the event that I do not have an opportunity to do so later. Accordingly, this book should be regarded as number 1 of ? volumes.[1] Whether there will be subsequent volumes will depend upon how long I live and what I achieve in the process.

Andrew I. Batavia
August 12, 2003 [the planned date of publication]

Helping to Complete Drew's Memoirs

Drew passed away on January 6, 2003, before he could complete and publish his memoirs, the target date for which had been August of that year. He had written fourteen chapters. I was approached to complete his work, but the writing was as perfect as it was unfinished. I didn't want to touch it, lest I adulterate it. And several family members could have stepped up to the task. So why get involved, more than a decade after his death, dredging up past grief, opening healed wounds, and unearthing new ones? What would be gained? These thoughts hopscotched through my mind.

I rationalized, as his younger brother by two and a half years, that I was the person (except for our mother) most privy to his forty-five-year life, from early childhood, when we shared a bedroom in Bensonhurst, to our final visit at his bedside in the ICU at Miami's Jackson Memorial Hospital in 2003.

But to be truthful, we were not particularly close as kids, and we did not interact except for teasing, rivalry, and physical fights. We did travel together on holiday trips to see our grandparents in Hallandale Beach, Florida, and frequented the same sleepaway camps, but even then I was never his confidant until shortly before his accident. Nevertheless, we had a common interest: We religiously tuned in to *The Tonight Show* starring Johnny Carson around bedtime on Drew's black-and-white twelve-inch TV. Following squabbles, however, he would turn the set away from my view. I would return the favor by pulling the plug on my eight-track player when a fight ensued. Such is the rivalry of brothers.

But there was tenderness, too. One night, at a rented summer house in upstate New York, while our parents were out, Drew climbed to the top of the refrigerator to fetch me a banana, my comfort food, to console me during a raging thunderstorm. But our relationship really began to cement shortly before Drew's accident. During his training for the upcoming Yonkers Marathon, we pounded the Westchester pavement together. As a teenager, he rounded up his friends and circled the village bully (every town had one) with their bicycles, making it clear that I was off his menu. And at one summer camp, I became his confidant. In short, he became my older brother.

And following his injury—during Drew's "mega-morphosis"—we kept in touch. I witnessed his rehab at Rusk, his move to Harvard, his parenting at "Bedlam," his tenure at FIU. And I stood as best man at his wedding. His circumstances swayed my choice of careers toward physical therapy. And as our careers in higher education crossed, we published together. Perhaps we're doing it once more.

Now, with more than a decade of distance since his death, I believe I have the clarity to offer a fair perspective of Drew's life. In doing so, I have uncovered a surprising amount about Drew, his life, and my relationship with him. I would like to believe, though I am by no means certain, that I shared at least a shred of DNA with him, a twin-like connectivity that could offer some special insight into his journey. Perhaps, though we were miles apart on the day of

Drew's accident, the burning crater I felt in the lining of my gut wasn't the mystery meat at camp.

In the end, what convinced me to finish Drew's memoirs was his deathbed wish that either his wife, Cheryl, or I do so. When Cheryl approached me with the project in the spring of 2015, I was astounded by the captivating prose of Drew's unfinished work, which had been found in his computer files. What a treasure of life experiences nearly lost. It must be published, I thought. And reading it is like having Drew back in our lives, as if I could turn back time, albeit temporarily.

Drew's writing has not been altered except for minor edits, use of a few pseudonyms where indicated, and some phrasing to reflect current disability language when he refers to others; historical information (publication excerpts, speeches, letters with quotes) remains unchanged. I penned the final ten chapters and provided commentary on several others, pulling from his publications, eulogies, holiday letters, family anecdotes, photographs, interviews, tenure files, letters, and my own memories. My contributions are noted with the heading "Mitchell Batavia, Brother." Cheryl, and my mother, Renée, were indispensable partners during this memoir project. They, along with other relatives and friends, provided anecdotes and documents for its completion. I am grateful to my wife, Evgenia, and son, Michael, for their patience during this year-long project. To preserve Drew's voice and get the publication out around the time of the ADA's twenty-fifth anniversary year, the family decided to publish this work on their own rather than use a traditional publisher, which might have had competing commercial interests.

Drew's memoirs are published as a lasting gift for his two children, his family and friends, and for a wider audience both within and outside the disability community, where

Drew's rich escapades might serve as a model for living fully, despite or perhaps because of his life in a wheelchair.

Mitchell Batavia
March 31, 2016

Acknowledgments

This book is dedicated, first and foremost, to my children, Joe and Katey. However, it is also dedicated to the other many, many wonderful people who have contributed in a positive manner to my life, who are mentioned by name throughout this book, as well as the few nasty, miserable people who tried unsuccessfully to hold me down, who will remain nameless. All of these people—the good, the bad, and the ugly—have contributed significantly to the very full experience of my life, and I am eternally grateful to each of them.

As always, I particularly appreciate the strong support of my entire family, including my wife, Cheryl; my parents, Renée and Gabriel; the other members of my family, Donna, Mitch, Genia, David, T.J., Ellen, and Clifford; and my extended family, Jeanine, Lauren, and Emily Drew. There is nothing as important as family, and even if it were possible to achieve great accomplishments without them, the reason for doing so would be greatly diminished.

A.I.B.

Part 1. The Full Experience

I can remember when I was very young thinking that irrespective of how my life unfolds, I just hope it is interesting. The one thing that I could not tolerate would be a boring life. I have what one might refer to as a "low threshold for boredom," a complicated way of saying I need constant stimulation. This attribute is a mixed blessing, in that it can motivate one to do many things with one's life, but it will not let you rest. When asked if I ever get tired after working on

I can remember when I was very young thinking that irrespective of how my life unfolds, I just hope it is interesting.

my computer for twelve or fourteen consecutive hours, six or seven days a week for several months during a busy period, I sometimes repeat the answer that my mother, from whom I apparently inherited this trait, gives: "I will have plenty of time to rest when I die."

In looking back at my youthful hope for an interesting life, I am reminded at this time of the now-famous Chinese curse that you should be very careful what you wish for lest it come true. In fact, I can hardly imagine a more interesting life. This is not because I am rich and famous, which I am not. It is not because I have achieved anything great, which I may or may not have done. It is mostly because I have been able to maintain a normal, and in some ways super-normal, life under circumstances that could often be considered adverse, despite many people telling me along the way that I could not.

Although my life has never been boring, it also has not always been easy or comfortable. Some of this difficulty and pain are portrayed in the following pages, which may exceed the comfort level of some readers. I hope that this is not the case, or if it is, I hope it does not deter people from reading on. I remember, after my injury, thinking that I would not allow this inconvenience to interfere with my ability to have an interesting life, and that I wanted to have "the full experience."

To me, the full experience meant that I would be able to experience all the joy and the pain associated with living in this world, just like anyone else. I do not want to be shielded from the pain. One of the worst aspects of disability is that some pain-in-the-ass people try to protect you from the realities of life, thinking you are too weak to take the pain. I am not weak, nor are most people with disabilities. You have to be strong to survive with a major disability in this world. As discussed in this part, I have survived and more.

Most important to me, I have had the full experience. Maybe, in some ways, I have had more than the full experience. I would not trade a day of it for anything, or switch my life with that of any other person.

Chapter 1. No Log Cabins in Brooklyn (or Yonkers)

In writing an American autobiography, it is always useful to be able to say that you were born in a log cabin or "in the house my father built." I was not born in a log cabin, and neither of my parents were in the construction business! As far as I know, there is not a single log cabin in Brooklyn, where I emerged on June 15, 1957. Despite this unfortunate deficit, I am very proud to be from Brooklyn, which has been the birthplace of a disproportionate number of very prominent and successful Americans. Sometimes, when my students do not understand something I have said in a lecture, I tell them that it is probably my Brooklyn accent. In actuality, if there is a trace of that dialect remaining, it is remarkable after years of living in California, Massachusetts, Virginia, Washington, DC, and Florida, but my Brooklyn roots remain important to me.

I was born in Beth-El Hospital (now Brookdale), which is admittedly not as good as a log cabin, but probably somewhat safer from a purely medical perspective. My parents tell me that they were dining at a Chinese restaurant when I rudely interrupted their meal with the unambiguous message that I was ready to come out. This may, in part, explain my lifelong love of Asian food, though I cannot verify this scientifically.

The frenetic taxi ride to the hospital may explain my phobia of the roads, though my car accident sixteen years later may also have something to do with this "irrational fear."

I thank God that I was born in this most important of the five boroughs of New York City to my family, and that we got out when we did.

Bad and Good Omens

If you are from Brooklyn, you no doubt noticed the year I was born—1957; if you are not from Brooklyn, you may not recognize the significance of that date. It turns out that being born in 1957 in Brooklyn was extremely poor timing, though it seems very unfair to hold me accountable in any way for the tragedy of that year. To paraphrase President Franklin D. Roosevelt, 1957 is "a date which will live in infamy," at least in Brooklyn. That was the year that the great Brooklyn Dodgers left the legendary Ebbets Field for Los Angeles, of all places. Few teams have ever been as dearly loved by their hometowns, and few hometowns have ever been as devastated by the departure of their team; some Brooklynites are still grieving over this today.

Some who are inclined toward soothsaying would contend that being born in 1957 was a very bad omen and that my life prospects would not be very great. Of course, at the age of only a few months, I was largely oblivious to this development. Still, even at that young age, one is no doubt affected by one's environment, and there were not a lot of happy people in Brooklyn that year. The exception to this general discontent was my family, who seemed very pleased with my arrival.

If asked to provide one single piece of advice to be successful in this world, I would say to choose your family very carefully. It seems ironic that such a key factor to success is largely out of the control of almost all of us. Interestingly, my own children had this choice when they were asked at the ages of six and four whether they wanted to leave their orphanage in Russia to join our family in the United States. Although I did not have this choice, luck had it that I was born into the most wonderful family in the world. Some readers may respectfully disagree with this conclusion, but they would be wrong.

Much as one gets points for being born in a log cabin, it appears highly desirable to be able to say that you are related in some way to the British royal family; bonus points apply for claiming direct kinship with the Queen of England. As far as I know, I am not related to any of these people in any way, nor do I understand why one would want to admit to such a relationship. My family came to this country from Russia and Poland three or four generations ago as Jewish immigrants from countries that did not enthusiastically embrace their diversity. Like many Americans, I do not know much about my ancestors, only that they must have been remarkably resilient and intelligent people to survive and escape the oppression of their native lands and to succeed in this country, which also did not enthusiastically embrace their diversity.

On my mother's side, I come from a long line of educators. My grandfather Joseph Hyman (whom my son, Joe, was named after), was the assistant principal of a vocational school in New York City. As such, he was responsible for disciplining some of the toughest kids in the Bronx, and he was a no-nonsense, old-school kind of guy. His parents, Bella and Abraham (for whom I received the *A* in my first name), came from Russia in the late nineteenth century and instilled a sense of social responsibility in their son. Grandpa Joe was the person who would inevitably organize social and charitable activities and had a real commitment to community service. At family gatherings and social functions, he was always prepared with a slightly risqué joke that began with several minutes of setup in English inevitably followed by a punch line in Yiddish, causing everyone to laugh hysterically, with the exception of me and my siblings. This taught me early the value of learning a foreign language, though Yiddish would not have been my first choice.

Joe Hyman married Anne Shradnick, who came to this country, from Russia to Ellis Island, at the age of two, and who must be one of the nicest people who has ever inhabited this Earth. I have never heard my Grandma Anne say a bad word about anybody. Even now, at the age of ninety-nine, with little short-term memory left, she is the most pleasant person you can imagine, and her eyes continue to light up whenever you say the name of Grandpa Joe. Anne was a housewife for most of her life, except when she worked as a secretary to a deaf man as a teenager, served as a volunteer during World War II, and helped Joe with his electrical business when he was getting his education. With her support, he ultimately received a bachelor's and a master's degree, and completed most of the requirements for a PhD (in the days that very few people had more than a high school diploma). Although being a housewife may sound trivial to some in this age of feminism, Anne Hyman was a true partner in the success of her husband and their family.

I have much less direct knowledge of my father's side of the family, because his father died before I was born, and I was only thirteen when his mother died, on my birthday and five days before my bar mitzvah.

Grandpa Isadore, who is the reason that my middle initial is *I*, was a businessman who sold women's apparel, which is most of what I know about him. If anyone is interested in how he got the name Batavia, the short answer is that we have no idea. Batavia is a popular name in the Netherlands, and the capital of the former Dutch colony of Indonesia, currently named Jakarta, was once named Batavia. Apparently, the name comes from the Batavi tribe that inhabited Holland in early times. The Jewish people wandered a lot throughout Europe, after getting kicked out of their countries every once in a while; we must have picked up the name somewhere along the way, possibly at Ellis Island, where officials had the prerogative to name you whatever inspired them at the moment. However we got the name, we are pleased with it; we could have done much worse than Batavia.

Grandma Mary, from whom my daughter, Katerina Marie, received her middle name, owned a small and barely profitable women's apparel store in Eastchester, New York, after moving the business from Harlem. Her most important achievement, at least from my perspective, was ensuring the survival of my father when he contracted polio at the age of three. Despite extremely limited financial resources, Mary did everything in her power to take my father to the very best health care practitioners of the day, including a chiropractor who helped him walk after many physicians could not. That effort, and the good fortune that the polio virus did not spread to the rest of his body, allowed him to live a normal life, walking with a substantial limp, and graduate from the City College of New York, which was regarded as the "Harvard of the Poor" at the time.

My father, Gabriel, is one of the best men I have ever known. It is impossible for me to summarize all the reasons that I feel this, but part of it has to do with his love of his family and his commitment to honesty and decency. Much of what he has taught me was conveyed less through words than through actions. Due largely to the circumstances of his family, having survived with little during the Great Depression, he chose to be a certified public accountant, which has to be the single most boring profession ever devised. In those days, the accounting profession did not entail all of the creativity of the current profession, which has given us such great things as the Enron and WorldCom fiascos. Back then, accounting entailed the honest but mind-numbing arithmetic of debits and credits; I remember vividly his dragging himself home after long, ten-hour days in his Manhattan office only to spend countless additional hours into the night during the dreaded tax season, and then to repeat the cycle the following day.

My father's favorite fictional character, Don Quixote, became a part of my inspiration to achieve a quest that may seem to some impossible

I saw my father as a cog in a horrible machine, which paid the bills but exacted an enormous human cost. He was, and is, a creative human being who was deprived of the opportunity to exercise his creativity. It is very gratifying that now, at age eighty-two, he is enjoying the expression of his creativity through his sculpture. I watched him suffer for years in an unrewarding career that took a toll on his health. I admired him for doing this for his family, but I vowed I would never let it happen to me. I would control my destiny to the fullest extent possible, and I would not work to ensure the fortunes of people less worthy than myself. Most important, I would find a way to ensure that my values would be reflected and my creativity would be applied in my chosen profession.

My father also gave me an empathy for the underdog, for whom he always rooted, and a recognition of the importance of a sense of mission. As a long-term fan of the world champion Boston Celtics, in a city in which being a Celtics fan was not very popular, I did not always follow his lead in rooting for underdogs; however, in my defense, I stuck with the Celts in the bad years as well as the good. (I am now an owner of the Celtics franchise as a result of my wife's purchasing me one share for my thirty-fifth birthday, a gift that keeps on giving, in that I receive a dividend check for $1.75 every year.) My father's favorite fictional character, Don Quixote, became a part of my inspiration to achieve a quest that may seem to some impossible. Although my father was never able to pursue his own quest, other than raising a wonderful family, he was able to instill that mentality in me. For this, I am eternally grateful.

My mother, Renée, is the single most important reason that I am alive now to write this.

I tend to take the long view, much the way certain Asian cultures do, that even if these things may not be achieved in a lifetime, they can be achieved in the next generation or the generation after that.

My mother, Renée, is the single most important reason that I am alive now to write this. She is the most remarkable woman I have ever known. Much as my Grandma Mary ensured the survival of my father, my mother ensured my survival by guaranteeing that every possible resource available in our society would be used to help me recover and live a normal life. Although she was a kindergarten teacher in New York City throughout her career, she became the most effective social worker that city had ever seen. Through her advocacy, New York State Vocational Rehabilitation Services was able to recognize my potential and finance my education at the University of California and Harvard Law School. Beyond all this, while dealing with all the trauma associated with my injury, she was able to hold the family together and take care of the needs of my younger siblings, Mitch and Donna, who were still adolescents at the time.

Finally, Mitch and Donna are the best brother and sister one could hope for in a lifetime. Mitch, my long-term roommate prior to going to college, is a member of the faculty of New York University. Donna is a professional on Wall Street with highly valued analytical skills. Both are very successful in their personal and professional lives. Although my parents were concerned that they might never settle down, they recently got married within a couple of months of each other. Donna married a talented photographer, David, at their beautiful lakeside summer home. Mitch got married at the famous Russian Tea Room in Manhattan to a beautiful Russian woman, Genia, thereby continuing the long Russian tradition of our family. Mitch and I have collaborated on several published articles together, including one on the therapeutic benefits of karaoke for people with quadriplegia and other disabilities.

Brooklyn Memories

To be honest, my memories of Brooklyn are somewhat murky at this point, in that my family left Brooklyn when I was nine years old. Still, they say that the first ten years of life are most formative, and whenever I am asked on a government form where I am from, I always write in

"Brooklyn." I may not sound like it anymore, but I will always be a Brooklyn boy, at least to some extent.

One of my very first memories was of the construction of the Verrazano-Narrows Bridge, the longest bridge of its kind in the world for a number of years. It was being built near our apartment on Shore Road in the Bay Ridge section of Brooklyn, which looked out at the water. We moved to the Bensonhurst section of Brooklyn when I was two years of age. Bensonhurst is a historical community that consisted largely of Jews and Italians at that time. I learned, many years later, that this community was the home of a fair number of middle-level Mafia members, which may explain why the trash was always picked up on time and there was relatively little petty street crime. I did not know anything about this at the time, in that my family always made our money the old-fashioned way—we earned it.

My best memories of Bensonhurst relate to a variety of smells. Those people who think that Brooklyn, or New York City in general, does not smell so good did not live there in the 1950s and 1960s. I remember vividly taking in remarkable scents of pizza and other ethnic foods when walking along the major avenues. However, these were not even as good as what you would smell when you entered my grandparents' apartment, which was several blocks away from our house. My Grandma Anne made the best stuffed cabbage that has ever been baked in the history of Jewish cooking. Every holiday, we would go there and feast on a variety of dishes, each of which was better than the last, and most of which no doubt continue to line my arteries to this day. Other favorite memories of Brooklyn include my grandparents' taking us to Coney Island, one of the first great amusement parks in this country.

Other Brooklyn memories were not as good. We lived on the bottom floor of a two-family house owned by an old married couple who lived upstairs. The best part of this house was the cherry tree that overhung from the neighbor's yard, giving us cherries for a good part of the year and proving that a tree can, in fact, grow in Brooklyn. Although I did not really understand what was happening in those early days, I always had a sense of tension from "the landlords," who were not always happy about the amount of noise my siblings and I sometimes made. I would occasionally have the unpleasant responsibility of conveying the monthly rent check to these people, who never gave any indication that they were pleased to see me (as opposed to the check, which they were pleased to see). To make matters worse, our part of the house was tiny and seemed even tinier when my sister, Donna, arrived in 1962. Fortunately, my parents had accumulated enough money for a down payment on a house soon thereafter, and we were able to leave Brooklyn.

Before we left, however, there was one other bad memory I had to take with me. This was really not a memory at all, but rather a perception that became a part of my reality, as well as that of my brother. Fortunately, there also was one other positive memory that largely counteracted it. In our little neighborhood, there were two large, looming presences—one very negative and one very positive.

The negative presence was that of Frankie,[1] some juvenile delinquent, apparently without a last name, who had developed a legendary reputation in our Brooklyn community. I am a little fuzzy on the facts forty years later; I believe that Frankie was known for killing and eating young children, or something like that. My brother and I, and hundreds of other Bensonhurst kids, lived in constant fear of being confronted by Frankie, although I had never met anyone who had actually been confronted by him. (Of course, if someone had been so confronted, the individual logically would have already been eaten and therefore unavailable to tell me about the confrontation.)

The positive presence was that of Sandy Koufax, the great Jewish Brooklyn Dodgers pitcher, who had grown up in Bensonhurst and who attended the same Jewish Community Center we attended. Koufax distinguished himself both on the field, with his brilliant pitching (including a perfect game), and off the field, by refusing to pitch the first game of the World Series because it was on Yom Kippur, the Jewish High Holy Day. Being from the same neighborhood as Sandy Koufax was in some way like being related to a great person, even better than being related to the Queen of England. Although I was never much of a baseball fan (having been personally responsible for the departure of the Dodgers), I still like the idea of being from the same place as Sandy Koufax.

In any event, we left Brooklyn before having the honor of meeting Frankie and well after Sandy had left at the time of my birth. I did meet several individuals who apparently were attempting to achieve Frankie's status. This may explain my lifelong contempt for bullies and my ongoing commitment to knock them down at every available opportunity. Heroes like Sandy Koufax, through their example, give you the resolve and courage to do so. I have his autographed picture on my office wall, close to my marathon number and Celtics stock certificate.

Lost and Found in Yonkers

We moved to Yonkers just before I entered the fourth grade. Yonkers is probably most famous as the setting of *Hello, Dolly!*, the corporate home of Otis Elevator (the largest elevator manufacturer in the country for many years), the place of a famous harness racetrack, and the home of Son of Sam (the serial murderer who distinguished himself in the annals of crime by following the instructions of his dog). More recently, the famous playwright Neil Simon wrote a play called *Lost in Yonkers,* which played on Broadway for a period of time.

I was also lost in Yonkers for a period of time. It is not that Yonkers was a bad place to grow up. In many ways, it was an ideal place. The neighborhood to which we moved was aesthetically beautiful, every house was unique architecturally (although all were made of bricks and stones, and there were no log cabins). I still enjoy driving through the old neighborhood whenever we are in New York. Our house, a three-story colonial on Crawford Street, was a wonderful home for about ten years of my life.

It was never difficult to find a pickup game of basketball or touch football in this Italian-Irish-Jewish neighborhood. In doing so, you inadvertently learned how to deal with people from other backgrounds who seemed to have an endless arsenal of ethnic slurs specifically tailored to address your particular situation. It made you feel very special knowing that they spent so much time and thought on your ethnicity. I was often referred to as a "good Jew," one of those backhanded compliments that warranted a similar retort on my part concerning their particular pedigree or the marital status of their parents at the time of their birth.

I later learned that, in considering where to move from Brooklyn, the other option my parents were contemplating was Long Island. Not being much of a manicured-lawn type of guy, suffice it to say that I am glad they chose Yonkers.

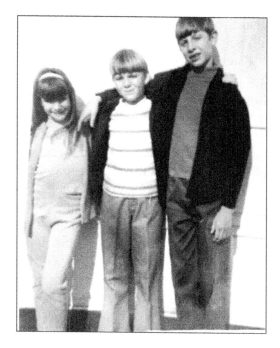

Donna, Mitch, and Drew posing in front of their Yonkers home soon after moving from Brooklyn [Left to Right].

So why was I lost? I was bored, and nothing is worse for me than being bored. In my mind, life was going to begin when I was on my own, which would begin in college. There was never a doubt in anyone's mind that I would be going to college and then become some kind of professional. I always received As in school, and I had two generations of college graduates in my family to serve as role models. The only question was which school I would attend and what field I would enter. In the meantime, I needed to do something to alleviate my boredom. Contrary to my nature, I resorted to the two traditional responses to this age-old dilemma: sports and girls.

My pursuit of sports primarily entailed joining the Lincoln High School track team. I had previously tried out for the basketball team, in two consecutive years, and was the last to be cut in each year. The fact that it was a very good team, ultimately reaching the county finals in my senior year, was little consolation. I tried out for track my sophomore year, with the substantial advantage of knowing that nobody ever gets cut from the track team. I became a decent, but not great, long-distance runner. I always had more potential than talent, and fate had it that there was not enough time for that potential to be realized. The highlight of my sports career was running the Yonkers Marathon, one of the first and most recognized in the country, in three hours and thirty minutes, a respectable time for a fifteen-year-old. I spent the following day in the bathtub. I still have my marathon number—349— hanging in my office. The marathon was in May 1973, three months before my injury; one of the things for which I am most grateful is that I did this before I became disabled.

Like most of my fellow students, my pursuit of girls was about as successful as my athletic career. That is, until one day in biology class. In an effort to demonstrate that chivalry was not dead, I offered to assist the girl in the next desk with the dissection of her frog, sensing that she was less than enthusiastic about doing this. I tell myself now that the fact that she was a beautiful blond girl in no way motivated this chivalry, but I cannot delude myself. In any event, over the year, Lisa and I became very close (and remain close by long-distance to this day). Our closeness was mostly platonic, which was more a result of my lack of guts than anything else, and I vowed to remedy this as soon as I returned from being away during the summer after our sophomore year. For reasons that were beyond the control of either of us, this was not to be.

Chapter 2. Preparation and Disaster

I was at the top of my game. I just celebrated my sixteenth birthday, completed my sophomore year of high school with pretty much straight As, finished my first marathon in good time, and had a very attractive girlfriend. I would be applying to some of the top schools in the country the next year, and I expected to be accepted by my top choices. The only thing I did not have was a job to pay for all the expenses I expected would be cropping up in the next year or so. I had no idea at the time what an impact my first job would have on my life.

Pursuing First Employment

In fact, I had never had a job. This was not because we were rich, which we were not. My family, with both my father and mother working, had an income that was average in our middle-class Yonkers community. We certainly had more than some, but much less than others, and I cannot remember a time in which money was not tight. However, my parents knew their priorities, and the top priority was for me to study hard and to maintain a good social life. They would not have allowed me to work during the school year if I had wanted to, and I gave no indication that I wanted to.

I do not like to think of myself as having been spoiled, but I suppose that must have been the way it appeared to some of my fellow students who did have to work part-time to help out their families. Some of them had a variety of jobs and consequently had some disposable income, which meant money in their pockets for things they wanted. This seemed to me to be a desirable thing.

For example, two small Italian cousins had a job in which they delivered betting sheets before the weekend, collecting the appropriate amount of money and paying off the winners at the beginning of the next week. This seemed like good work, if you could get it, which you could not unless you had the right family connections. Nepotism is a bad thing! I am not sure whether I thought through my jealousy of these guys; although this did not appear to be a very difficult job, a single arithmetic miscalculation could result in several broken bones.

The concept of having disposable income was very powerful, however, and my parents' prohibition of employment did not extend to summer work. One day, I went to school and saw a tiny notice on the bulletin board that said simply: "Job in summer camp. Call xxx-xxx-xxxx." I thought to myself, This is something that I am actually capable of doing. Along with my brother and sister, I had gone to summer camp for a number of years. I knew basically what a counselor was required to do, and I could do it. I went home and called the number.

The live voice on the other end of the line said something like, "Thank you for calling." Then the person asked if I was aware that this is a camp for children with severe intellectual disabilities. All of a sudden, I developed a distinct stutter that I never knew I had, and hung up the telephone fairly abruptly. I never really thought about working with anyone with severe disabilities before, and working with children with severe intellectual disabilities did not seem as easy as serving as an assistant bookie.

But then I thought about it for a while. I really was not qualified to do anything, and a "normal camp" would probably not hire a sixteen-year-old boy, which was basically what I was. Then I started thinking that this could actually be the first important thing I had ever done. And it certainly did not sound boring. I decided to call the number again, this time better prepared for the conversation.

The Question of Fate

In the previous chapter, I use the term "fate" in stating that I would not be able to complete some of the things I started in high school. The notion that all things are preordained, and therefore out of our control, is somewhat offensive to me. It really takes away the whole purpose in living, because whatever you think you've chosen to do actually would have been predetermined by fate. So whether or not we are destined by our fate, I choose to reject this notion. (Of course, I recognize that my choice not to recognize fate itself may be dictated by my fate, if I'm wrong about this.)

In any event, while I do not believe that my every action is determined by fate, I do believe that certain things in life are meant to be. I believe that I was meant to work at Camp Lee Mar in the summer of 1973. I believe that my experience that summer would help prepare me for the rest of my life. Of course, I did not know or believe these things at that time. Basically, what I knew was that I needed a summer job, and this one was probably the only one I could get. If I could get it!

So I dialed the number again. And I set up a tentative interview. And I told my parents about it, wondering how they would react. After some minor initial shock, they were thrilled that I was finally getting off my butt and earning my own way. I say this only somewhat facetiously, in that I do think they were pleased that I had taken the initiative to find a summer job. I also think they were pleased with my choice, which was a job entailing significant responsibility.

There was still one small matter: getting the job. I honestly cannot remember the interview, or even if there was a face-to-face interview. I am sure that there was some type of interview by the camp director, Lee Morrone, one of the most respected people in the area of intellectual disability at the time and the mother of a child with an intellectual disability. Apparently, the interview must have gone well, because I got the job. I was particularly proud of this, in that it was my very first job and at age sixteen I was going to be the youngest counselor at a camp for kids with intellectual disabilities. Whether my getting this job was a matter of fate, I will leave to you.

My Best Summer Ever

I mentioned earlier that I spent much of my youth waiting for it to end. And this summer was as close as I had come to being on my own. Of course, there was still plenty of adult supervision, but it was a different type of supervision than I had experienced previously. The adult who would become closest to me was Bob Peters. Bob was a legend at the camp. He was a full-time teacher of children with intellectual disabilities during the year, who spent his summers as a counselor at the camp for many years. I am sure that he was assigned as a senior counselor of our group, in large part, because Lee wanted to be sure I had appropriate adult supervision, and he was the best.

I can still remember the first week of camp in early July 1973. The counselors and other staff arrived the week before the kids. The administration held marathon meetings with the counselors, briefing us on every aspect of every camper, not just the campers assigned to our groups. Throughout the summer, each of us would work, in some way, with each and every camper. We needed to know their functional levels, medical conditions, medications, and other personal characteristics. Medical conditions were particularly important, because many of these children had multiple disabilities; for example, many of them also had epilepsy and required medications to control their seizures, which could be life-threatening.

I said that this was a camp for children with intellectual disabilities. Well, some of these "children" were about ten years older than I was and had more hair on their chests than I had on my entire body. The fact that their mental ages ranged from between seven and ten still did not reduce the initial shock of seeing them. At times throughout the summer, I had night duty, in which it was my responsibility to wake up some of these big guys very gingerly in the middle of the night to give them their antiseizure medications; if one were to wake one of them too abruptly, it could trigger an epileptic seizure, in which case I would have to basically wrestle the camper down to the ground and try to make sure that he did not swallow his tongue, which would be a bad thing.

The thought of engaging in a midnight wrestling match with someone twice my weight and three times my strength was not that appealing to me. However, this is what I was envisioning as we were being briefed in the first week. Fortunately, I never had to deal directly with a major seizure, and I actually enjoyed working with these older campers very much. At one point in the summer, I was responsible for teaching sex education to these guys, which was extremely amusing. They seemed particularly fixated on the significance of the navel, on which we spent a disproportionate amount of time, considering its limited importance. However, during this first week, before I met them, it was starting to become apparent that this was some very serious business, particularly for a sixteen-year-old who was just learning to take care of himself.

This is not to suggest that every minute of the first week was all business. There was a fair amount of opportunity to meet the other counselors and staff members, who were truly a remarkable group of people. These were individuals who were deeply dedicated to their work, which paid more in personal fulfillment than financial enrichment. Among the most common topics of conversation was: "When is Bob going to get here?" I heard every Bob Peters story that the many returning counselors had to tell, and most of them came back year after year. It was clear to me that this was a very remarkable person and teacher. I was not disappointed when I finally met him later in the week. He taught me everything I needed to know, and we remain friends to this day.

Among the staff members were a group of waitresses, who were around my age, one of whom was more attractive than the next. During the off hours, we got to see a lot of each other and got to know each other fairly well in a brief period of time. In some ways, we really saw a lot of each other, in that the camp had one communal shower for staff, and when you were showering, it was not at all unusual for a young lady to be in the next stall. While everyone seemed very comfortable with this arrangement, I was a little concerned about getting somewhat overstimulated, if you get my meaning. Sensing my anxiety over this, the head waitress comforted me by saying, "Don't worry, my girls have seen them up, down, and moving."

I do not mean to suggest that this was like Sodom and Gomorrah, with orgies occurring in the hallways, which was certainly not the case, but there was a fair amount of coupling up throughout the summer. This sexually charged atmosphere was particularly challenging to a person who was approaching his physiological sexual peak (which I subsequently learned occurs at about nineteen years of age for males) and who was trying to focus on learning his responsibilities. Fortunately and unfortunately, I was not exempt from all of this hyperhormonal activity, and I developed some experience that summer. In an attempt to alleviate my guilt over Lisa, I tried to convince myself that I was getting this experience for her, which demonstrates definitively that all men are, in fact, pigs.

This leads me to one episode of which I am not particularly proud. Apparently, as a result of one of these liaisons with a young lady, I managed to neglect some of my responsibilities at one point early in the summer. I really cannot recall the specifics, but I remember the consequences very well. The camp administration learned about this, and I was taken by Lee to the proverbial woodshed.

I had never been reprimanded for anything before at any time in my life, in part because I had never done anything wrong (with the possible exception of going to a Grateful Dead concert that ended in the middle of the night without having told my parents when it would be over, which they did not appreciate very much). As long as I can remember, everyone had always told me how mature I was for my age. They told me this at every age, which really started to get old after a while. For the first time, I was being told that I was immature, which was somewhat refreshing for a change, though Lee really let me have it verbally. I was not about to be irresponsible again, and there were no further problems that summer.

In my defense, I think everybody has a time in which they go a little wild, typically during the first year of college, and I was being somewhat precocious in my responsibility. Of course, this is much less a justification than an excuse, and it is a fairly lame excuse. There is actually no good excuse for what I did, because these kids really depended on every one of us, and a single mistake could have been fatal.

My Utopian Preparation

When the campers finally got there, I went through a transformation. I think that at that moment I became an adult. Partly as a result of Lee's reprimand, and largely as a result of the enormous responsibility that I felt the moment I saw them, I was changed. I was also the happiest I had ever been. My happiness was in part the result of my transformation to early adulthood and the recognition that I was finally on my own.

But my happiness was even more a result of being a part of something much greater than myself. It was a result of being a part of the closest thing I would ever get to a utopian society. Everyone was there for the kids. These kids had more problems on a daily basis than I had experienced in my entire life. Yet they were happy. They were more than happy; they were filled with joy. They were sometimes frustrated with their limitations, but they learned to deal with it, and they taught me patience in doing so.

Most important, there was never any pettiness on the part of anyone. I am not sure whether this was because these people were just not inclined toward pettiness (which I am sure was a lot of it), or because there was just not enough time or energy for people to be petty, or because people were just too happy to engage in such nonsense, but it was wonderful.

I did not know it at the time, but the summer would be the best possible preparation for the challenges I would face for the rest of my life. I had never really known a person with a disability before. The closest I had ever gotten to knowing such a person was my own father, but he just had a severe limp from his childhood polio, which resulted in a lot of pain but did not really limit his functioning. Now I knew an entire camp of people with disabilities. I would never trade the disability that I would acquire with that of any of the kids in this camp. Yet they dealt with it with dignity, courage, and joy. They will never know how much the few weeks I spent with them helped me for the next thirty years. That long period of time began toward the end of that summer, in one split second.

Disaster

One day toward the end of the camp season, on August 12, 1973, two of the waitresses and I decided to take our day off together and to go to the resort town of Monticello, New York. We had only one day off a week, and by that day we really needed to get away. Unfortunately, none of us had a car or even drove, so we decided to hitchhike. Now, I can just see the disapproving looks on some of your faces: How could we be so stupid as to hitchhike? Although I certainly do not contest that this was a stupid thing to do, in those days a lot of people hitchhiked. Unlike the situation now, in which hitchhikers occasionally have their heads stored in a bottle in some psychopath's refrigerator, this was before such horror stories.

Monticello was about a half hour or so away from Lackawaxen, Pennsylvania, where the camp was located. Somehow, we were able to get there, and we had a nice day. As the day progressed, however, clouds started rolling in, and it began to rain. We had to work the next day, so we started hitching to get a ride home. Thanks to the physical attractiveness of my traveling companions, we were able to do so in short order. A sports car stopped and took us in. The driver was a young man, and his dog was in the front passenger seat. The girls and I got in the backseat, and, being the gentleman that I was, I sat in the middle.

That is the last thing I remember on that day. Everything else was related to me by others after the fact. Apparently, the driver had been drinking or taking drugs, which we did not know when we got in his car, and he tumbled the car in the rainstorm. There were no seat belts in the backseat; consequently, the two girls smashed into the bucket seats in front of them, breaking a nose and arm, respectively. Being in the middle, I had no bucket seat in front of me, and I proceeded to fly through the windshield, ending up outside of the car. The driver had acquired a small scratch under his eye and lost his dog. I had broken my neck.

Commentary: Preparation for a Life Extraordinary
/Mitchell Batavia, Brother/

The accident—no one saw it coming. The best way Drew could have prepared for it, short of wearing body armor or lobbying for rear-center seat belts, was joining his high school track team. He had been cut from basketball tryouts, which likely broke his heart, but track strengthened it. And his training for the Yonkers Marathon he completed in the pouring rain at the age of fifteen put him in the finest physical condition of his life, three months before it was almost taken from him. Without this rigorous training, recovery from his injuries may have been tenuous.

One of the great mysteries about Drew, however, was not that he survived—though he almost didn't—but that he, despite or perhaps because of his quadriplegia, had such an extraordinary life. By all accounts, there was no prescience, no warning; his childhood was typical if not nondescript. He grew up in an average middle-class community, attended a garden-variety suburban high school, and dwelled in a silly-sounding city, Yonkers. We even had the typical sibling bantering at home. I would proceed to call him names that underscored his jutting nose or his tinseled braces; he would retaliate, wrestling me supine over one of our unattached bunk beds and taking playful shots to my shoulder. When our family occasionally sojourned to our favorite neighborhood Chinese restaurant, Jade Garden on Jerome Avenue in the Bronx, the menu choices would always be arranged in two columns, column A and column B. I don't recall the significance of the columns—one may have had more pricey chef specials. In any case, Drew would be on top of me and query, "Do you like one from column A or one from column B?" Of course, the "one" referred not to a dish, but to a punch, a jab executed tangentially across the outer rim of my bony left shoulder, a sting that lingered. I must confess, it was good fun.

But aside from the banter, Drew was a gentleman, as evidenced by his chivalrous act of sitting in the middle of the backseat, over the hump of the doomed Toyota. He was a model kid, a conformist. He was also quite reserved. In fact, Drew was so quiet as a child that our mother enrolled him in an elocution class to improve his expression and speech when he was about eight years old. For his final project, he was to present a speech in front of an audience—but he froze and said nothing. I mention this because this behavior is in stark contrast to the nonconforming, vociferous, activist role he later adopted, when not even a speech before the Supreme Court of the United States would rattle him. At conferences, Drew was known to give speeches of more than twenty minutes without using notes.

And Drew was well educated. He grew up in a Jewish family that placed heavy emphasis on learning. I remember my mother tenaciously drilling him in math in our Bensonhurst kitchen when he was seven or eight years old. She was a kindergarten teacher; her father, an assistant principal in a vocational school; and his father, a rabbi, a leader, and a scholar in his Brooklyn community: a lineage of teachers. And then there was our father, who was palpably intelligent and would have made a fabulous physician but chose a career in accounting, an occupation that can be conducted from a seated position, to accommodate polio scars from childhood. Although taciturn, whenever Dad offered advice (often on finances) it was piercingly wise and expressed in just the right number of words, no more and no less. Drew was surrounded by smart people.

All of this points to a childhood upbringing with good prospects for Drew—but an overly confident, Ivy League-trained, nonconforming activist? No one anticipated this. And the notion that he achieved more in his lifetime with only 10 percent of his body, and in half the time that most nondisabled persons could muster, was, well, somewhat baffling.

And while all this makes Drew sound like a saint, this was not completely true; there was just less to legitimately pick on. He did have strong, fairly unyielding opinions about most things (Shall we say opinionated?) and was less empathetic to others, or at least to me, in less dire situations than himself—which was practically everyone! My progressive hearing loss, a delightful trait passed along in our family, for example, did not lend itself to his sympathetic ear. Drew also set high standards for himself and held everyone else to those same heights. So if those who worked with Drew didn't pull their weight on a project, Drew would just finish the job himself rather than remediate or provide mentorship; personnel development was not his strong suit. Nevertheless, he did encourage others. Finally, Drew's taste in art was somewhat questionable; he had a strong affinity for kitsch. But this is just to say that no one is perfect.

Of course, I can conjure up explanations for his success. One theory is that, like me, he was a "late bloomer"—a term I abhor—someone who needed a bit more time to "steady his feet" and fully develop his potential. As if eventually your brain will mature, your nerve impulses will conduct faster, and you will catch up with the others. But I rejected this theory. First, it is patronizing; second, it's nonscience; and chiefly, I have evidence to discount it. As a younger brother who shared a bedroom with him, I, during weak moments, alone and curious, would shuffle through his dresser drawers to see what I could borrow. And what I discovered was striking. I came across a ninth-grade book report. The writing assignment was so well inked, constructed, and argued that it could not have possibly been written by someone in our family at such a young age. Perhaps it was his use of transitional words ("moreover," "furthermore," "along the same lines"), or maybe it was his use of contrasts ("neither wealth nor poverty"). He seemed in high school to already be a gifted author, with the concomitant talent of persuasion.

Still another reason I reject the late bloomer theory is my mother's recollection of a high school teacher-parent conference she attended with Drew prior to his accident. The encounter went something like this: "Did you know your son is a math genius?" My mom was both speechless and clueless. Drew clearly did not bloom late, just quietly.

A second explanation for his success is what I call the Theory of Forced Use, that without the use of his body and all its attending distractions (sports, driving, happy hours), he was forced to turn inward, toward his own mind, perhaps gaining special knowledge in the same way a person who is blind can feel. This may also explain his increased assertiveness following the accident, a trait one must rely on to survive quadriplegia. If he didn't speak up, how would he get things? For example, when his power chair was too feeble to make it up the hills of the UC Berkeley campus, he had to ask others to push him to class. Nevertheless, while this theory of forced use is entirely possible, I know scores of individuals who do not flourish despite bodily infirmities.

Still a third theory, which I am inclined to believe when I have no other, is that we were simply unrelated. I call this the Baby Stalk Theory or, alternatively, the Alien Implantation Hypothesis. He belonged to some other family but was left at our front stoop as a newborn. Although attractive, this explanation is unlikely. For one thing, family resemblance hints at a shared genetic footprint. Also, our knees cracked similarly when we squatted, and we both suffered from the same pattern of acid indigestion when stressed. More compellingly, our senses of humor were too similar to be coincidental. All we would have to do is glance at each other to read a punch line. Once, while watching a science fiction movie on television as kids, we witnessed a menacing, tower-size mud-man fall to the ground in pieces. I don't recall why it was so funny, but at the time, we were on the floor, gasping with laughter. His sense of humor also carried over after his injury. When he went off to college, he would dress up for Halloween. One year, he was a half-man/half-woman. Another year, at a professional conference in New Orleans, he dressed as a crayfish during Mardi Gras. Then there was the time he sent John Miller, a friend and naval officer who wore his hair razor-short, a gag gift of a cap with an attached ponytail. Drew knew when to be serious and when to be playful. His sense of humor ultimately contributed to his charm.

But beyond charm, Drew worked harder than most people, sitting up and clocking in ten- to-fourteen-hour days at the office, and then some on weekends. His wife, Cheryl, shared a story Drew told her about counting on the incompetence of others.

He said that most people are pretty lazy, and that he had overcome his disability and succeeded by working harder than most people are willing to work. When he arrived at Harvard Law School, he found himself in the company of other bright people who were equally motivated and did not have his physical limitations. He said that was the first time he really felt the impact of his disability on his efforts to excel.

And then there was preparation. Drew found his true life's work helping the disability community, and I believe that he, more than anyone else on this planet, was best suited to carry out this mission because of his qualifications. His training in law, economics, and health policy research, and his experiences in government and as a wheelchair user, made it so. He became a juggernaut in the disability rights movement.

But whatever the ultimate reason for Drew's success, he seemed to evolve from an unassertive, bright, conforming teenager into a dogged, visionary, hyperconfident activist with a penchant for adventure after he broke his neck. Like a weakened dam yielding to torrential water currents, Drew exploded into his new disability world after his injury, helping to give his community options, more access to public spaces, more hiring protections, fewer health care coverage exclusions. But conditions had to be right. First Drew had to become a person with a disability.

Chapter 3. My Acute Recovery

If your mother is anything like my mother, you have heard several thousand times in your life that you should not do any of a variety of risky things, "or you will break your neck!" It turns out that this is pretty good advice. Breaking your neck is not nearly as fun as it sounds. Most people who know anything about these matters immediately think that the person who has broken his or her neck will not be able to walk anymore, which they inevitably say in a tragic tone of voice.

If your mother is anything like my mother, you have heard several thousand times in your life that you should not do any of a variety of risky things, "or you will break your neck!"

Please believe me: If you break your neck, not being able to walk is the least of your problems. Virtually every system in the body is impacted dramatically by such a traumatic event. A broken neck has implications for every voluntary function and many involuntary ones, including the ability to feed oneself, bathe oneself, or even go to the bathroom independently. Had I known these things at the time that I flew through the windshield, I may have reconsidered doing so.

Initial Survival

The first order of business when you break your neck is to make sure that you continue breathing. Breathing is very important because when you stop doing it, oxygen is rapidly depleted from such key organs as your brain, and your life expectancy diminishes very rapidly. When I broke my neck, for some reason, breathing was never a major issue. I was very fortunate in that regard, as many people who break their necks struggle for breath initially and are routinely given tracheotomies (surgically cutting an opening in the trachea) and placed on ventilators, at least temporarily. Many of my friends bear the scars of this procedure, which I am just as happy not to have had. I have other scars instead.

I am particularly fortunate, although I really did not know it at the time, that the injury to my spinal cord was not slightly higher than it was. There are seven cervical vertebrae in the neck, and the higher your spinal cord is severed, the greater your level of paralysis, generally speaking. My spinal cord was severed quite high, between the second, third, and fourth cervical vertebrae. Due to my level of injury, I was paralyzed from below my shoulders, and half of my diaphragm is paralyzed.

If my injury had been an iota higher, my entire diaphragm would have been paralyzed, and I probably would have had to be on a ventilator permanently, much like Christopher Reeve about twenty years later. Back when I was injured, in 1973, very few people with that level of injury survived, and I would probably not be around to write this now.

The Rural Hospital

Soon after I was expelled from the car, an ambulance came to the scene of the accident. I have no recollection of this at all, as I was unconscious at the time. I was taken to a relatively small, rural hospital in upstate New York, where they did their best to stabilize my badly broken spine, though they were really not equipped to deal with the complexity of my situation. My parents had received the nightmare telephone call that no parent ever wants to get and drove upstate to the hospital. It was fortunate that they arrived safely, given their level of anxiety during the trip.

When they arrived, they were told that my situation was not good. They were told that I probably would not live, and even if I did my life prospects would be miserable. They were given two options. They could either keep me in that rural facility, where I would almost certainly die due to the lack of necessary expertise. Alternatively, they could authorize the transportation to a major medical center in New York City, in which case I would almost certainly die in transit due to the instability of my neck. They chose the trip to New York, which was the right choice.

I am not sure precisely when I regained consciousness. My first distinct recollection of being conscious was seeing my parents in the ambulance with me, though it is possible that I may have come to for periods of time in the rural hospital. I knew that something very bad had happened, and that I was not in good shape. However, I do not believe my mind allowed itself to realize that I was paralyzed. I did not acknowledge how badly I was injured until after I had arrived in New York. For the first time in my life, when he thought I was not looking, I saw my grandfather—the tough, stoic, mustached man I had always known—cry. This could not be a good sign.

In any event, I managed to survive the ambulance trip, and I was transported to the Montefiore Medical Center in the Bronx. This was one of the top tertiary-care medical centers in the country, and it gave me about as good a chance of survival as anyone in my condition.

Recovery at Montefiore

My neurosurgeon at Montefiore, a Dr. Ruben, was reputed to be one of the best in the country. He stabilized my spine in the traditional manner, in which he drilled a small hole in each side of my skull and thereby attached a traction device, called tongs, designed to keep my neck stable for a sufficient period of time for my neck bones to heal. To me, you have not lived until your head has been used as the equivalent of a two-by-four.

Many people who break their necks have fusion operations, whereby the surgeon fuses the bones together using heat. Unfortunately and fortunately, I was not able to have this procedure, because my neck was too unstable. This was unfortunate because it necessitated that I stay in the traction for a very long period of time, approximately three months. It was fortunate in that people who have fusion surgery often have a fairly limited range of motion in their necks for the rest of their lives. I told the doctor that, if he did this, I wanted him to install ball bearings in my neck so that I could turn it 360 degrees. He was not amused. In any event, I never had the procedure with or without ball bearings, and I can now move my neck fully, but not quite 360 degrees.

In looking back at my period of acute recovery, the word that immediately comes to mind is "torture." It really entailed a prolonged series of different tortures, which were very difficult to endure. Part of the torture was simply a matter of waiting for endless, boring hours while new calcium was being deposited ever so slowly, causing the fractured bones in my neck to heal. During this period, at different times, the hospital sent in three different psychologists to help me cope with my injuries. Each psychologist had his own special philosophy and clinical orientation.

The first psychologist told me that I needed to come to terms with the fact that I would be disabled for the remainder of my life, and therefore the sooner I accepted this reality, the better. The second psychologist told me that I needed to fight this thing, and that I should never accept my limitations. The third psychologist asked me whether there was anything I needed. I told him that I needed a small TV set for when I was lying on my stomach, so that I could have a diversion from what his colleagues were telling me. This fifty-dollar TV set was far more valuable than either of the first two psychologists. Needless to say, the third psychologist was my favorite.

A Variety of Tortures

Much of the torture of my acute recovery related directly to my physical circumstances. Simply recuperating from the initial injury was painful enough. But often the treatment was as uncomfortable as the underlying impairment. Having the tongs in my head for almost three months was almost unbearable. They were not able to bathe me adequately, and consequently my head always itched. Also, I looked a little like Frankenstein's monster, with those things sticking out of my head. My parents would not let me see a mirror for a long time, thinking that it would scare me.

But the worst thing was the Circ-O-Lectric bed, which I am convinced is a modern version of some medieval torture device. The purpose of this device is to avoid bedsores, technically known as decubitus ulcers. Bedsores are basically breakdowns of the skin resulting from the physical pressure between the external environment and the individual's bony prominences, particularly on the hips and buttocks. While all people experience such pressure on their skin, most are able to feel this pressure and shift their weight away from it. This is why people who are nondisabled constantly shift their positions throughout the night, when they are sleeping, and during the day, when they are sitting.

Because people with spinal cord injuries, such as me, are not able to feel the pressure—and even if we could feel it, could not shift our weight to reduce it—we are highly susceptible to bedsores. These are nasty things; if they get bad enough, they can bleed, become infected, and even become life-threatening. Fortunately, mine have never gotten that bad. However, like all people with quadriplegia, I have had problems with bedsores and have spent my share of time limited to bed rest in efforts to keep off the sore areas. This is often the only way they can heal.

The Circ-O-Lectric bed was designed to shift the position of the user so as to avoid the accumulation of undue pressure on the bones that can cause bedsores. It basically consists of two large circular hoops that stand parallel to each other, with a bed in between them. The patient is actually sandwiched between two mattresses, one on top and one on bottom. Every two hours or so, the operator of the bed presses a button, which electronically makes the bed rotate forward or backward, depending upon whether the individual is being placed on his stomach or his back. For about three months, I was moved in this manner—from my stomach to my back to my stomach to my back, and on and on—every two hours of every day, including throughout the night. Whenever I was to be rotated from my stomach to my back, the piece of the bed behind my head would have to be secured so that my head would have support.

I remember one time in the middle of the night, around 2 a.m., my nurse pressed the button and started the process by which the bed would start rotating backward. As my head was rising to about ninety degrees, I started feeling for the piece behind my head. At one point, although I was only halfway awake, I shouted "Stop!!!" The nurse had forgotten to secure the back piece. Fortunately, she stopped pressing the button; if she had continued to press for a few more seconds, I would have continued rotating backward and my neck would have snapped, either killing me instantly or at least setting me back several months. I had a different nurse the following day, but I never slept soundly again after this incident.

At one point during my prolonged relationship with my Circ-O-Lectric bed, I learned that I should be very happy to have it, because it is substantially better than the previous technology it replaced, the dreaded Stryker frame. Rather than rotating forward and backward, the patient was rotated sideways, from left to right, thereby achieving the same result as the Circ-O-Lectric bed in which the individual would go from stomach to back to stomach to back. However, because this device apparently predated the discovery of electricity, everything had to be done manually, which required at least two people.

Before flipping the patient sideways, the nurses would have to screw the top piece into place. Every once in a while, this process did not take, and the patient would fall to the floor. I now have a vague recollection of being in one of these things for a brief period of time at the rural hospital, which gave me a greater appreciation of the Circ-O-Lectric bed. Only now do I have a full understanding of how this bed saved me from the agony of permanent bedsores that have plagued many of my friends. Yet I did not understand these things at that time; all that I knew was that I was being tortured by technology on a daily basis.

Good Docs and Not-as-Good Docs

To make matters worse, every once in a while, some doctor would come into my room and stick me in the forehead with a pin. Unless you are personally inclined toward sadism, you might ask why a member of the medical profession would engage in such behavior. Inevitably, directly after doing this, the physician would ask me the essential question, "What percentage of feeling would you say this is?" Inevitably, I would respond by saying, "A hundred percent, you sadistic SOB!"

The point of this peculiar ritual was apparently to provide insight into my level of physical sensation to the physician and numerous medical students, who appeared to be there with a primary purpose of looking at my naked body. The stated objective was to compare the full feeling in those parts of my body that were not paralyzed, such as my forehead, with the less than full feeling in other parts of my body, which was treated much like a giant pincushion. Once I figured out this game, whenever a doctor would enter my room, I would tell him, "Let's just agree at the outset that the feeling in my forehead and everywhere else in my body above my shoulders is 100 percent."

Not all of my doctors were schmucks, fortunately. There are two in particular whom I will remember for the rest of my life for the positive things that they did for me: Dr. Golash and Dr. Kessel. I am not certain of the spelling of their names, and I do not know their first names, but these two young residents made a major difference for me. Toward the end of my three-month stay at the Montefiore Medical Center, I was told that I would soon be able to have the tongs taken out of my head and I could then leave the Circ-O-Lectric bed. Although I would have to wear a neck brace for a period of time, this seemed like heaven compared with what I had been through.

However, when the time came to take the tongs out, there was one last barrier. I needed to have a waterbed in my room to replace the Circ-O-Lectric bed. Waterbeds are extremely effective at reducing pressure and thereby preventing bedsores, and my senior physicians would not have me removed from the Circ-O-Lectric bed until the waterbed was available. For some reason, however, getting this bed was an almost impossible task. I told these residents that, if I did not get these things out of my head, I was going to explode. This was apparently the right thing to say, because neither of them had had a patient blow up on them before, and they particularly did not want this to happen on their shift (which, I imagine, would have entailed a lot of paperwork).

In the next twenty-four-hour period, these two young doctors worked virtually nonstop to ensure that the bed arrived, my tongs were removed, and I was transferred to the new bed in my new neck brace. Never in my life did I think that I would be so happy to have a neck brace. If Dr. Golash or Dr. Kessel read this, or if it is brought to their attention, I hope that they will contact me so that I can thank them personally for this. The fact that I remember their names after all these years should be a message to doctors that we appreciate their efforts when they go out of their way to help their patients.

Support and Release

These two physicians are not the only people to whom I owe a debt of gratitude. I also received enormous support from my family members and friends during this period. It would be impossible to ever pay back this debt or even acknowledge all the people to whom I owe it, in part because I was in such bad shape at the time that I was not even fully cognizant of all the people who provided such moral support. Yet, at some level, I felt all of it, and it made a big difference.

One person who deserves special mention, however, is my uncle Edgar Brush, who sent me a get-well card every single day that I was in the hospital that year. If you ever want to do something that really makes a difference in somebody's life, try doing this. He also wrote to my favorite basketball player, John Havlicek, the great Celtics star, who sent me an autographed picture. (I was somewhat embarrassed that later in the year I received two more signed pictures from him, because some of my other friends had the same idea, which is a tribute both to them and to Havlicek.)

My aunt Muriel, who was Ed's wife and my dad's younger sister, volunteered to stay with me to give my parents a break. Many friends dropped by later, often bearing gifts, all of which were truly appreciated. I believe that such support was as important to my recovery as the excellent medical care I received. One visitor who was not welcome was the driver who caused my injury; he had caused immeasurable suffering, and I asked the nursing staff to send him away. I had been warned that his attorney could advise him to drop by, and I wanted no part of this.

Once my neck was stabilized, I was ready to leave the hospital to go to a rehabilitation center so that I could prepare for the rest of my life. Unfortunately, there was one last impediment. The most respected rehabilitation hospital in the

United States at that time was Dr. Howard Rusk's Institute for Rehabilitation Medicine in Manhattan. My family wanted me to go to Rusk; unfortunately, there was a long waiting list. To this day, I do not know how I got into Rusk. I remember hearing, at one point, that the father of one of my friends had certain "connections." If this is the case, I certainly appreciate it, though I am hoping that no hospital administrator woke up in his bed one day with the detached head of his favorite pet. In any event, the next thing I knew, I was being transported by ambulance to Rusk.

Commentary: The Hospitalization
/Mitchell Batavia, Brother/

Montefiore is a massive urban medical metropolis in the North Bronx, well versed in handling the ravages of unstable neck bones and sliced spinal cords in persons who would be referred to as having tetraplegia (or quadriplegia), that is, all four limbs paralyzed. Drew could move and feel sensation only from the shoulders up. I was given Valium when my mom broke the news to me while being picked up from sleepaway camp at age thirteen. The pill persuaded my body to take a vacation and that life was dandy, when in fact it was not. It was that same summer of the accident when I made my first visit to Montefiore. I don't recall if it was day or night; there were no windows on the ward. I remember three things: Drew's single-occupancy room; the hallway, which was white, deserted, and sterile; and the recreational room used by patients who could make it out of their beds.

Of course, entering Drew's room and dealing with his tragedy was only compounded by my own guilt that I may have somehow, through magical thinking, contributed to his downfall. Earlier that year, my family was celebrating my bar mitzvah down in Orlando's Disney World. At a medieval exhibit of devices used to punish people through public humiliation, I took a snapshot of Drew posing in a pillory, a hinged wooden device with holes for restraining head and hands. I was involved in photography at the time, had set up a dark room in our basement, and even developed prints myself, and I developed the pillory photograph. Sometime later that year, Drew and I got into a fight over something he was looking for. He asked if I knew where it was, in what I felt was an accusatory tone. Understandably, he did not care for my reply and bulldozed me into a wall. In a rage, I took the pillory photograph and ripped it in half, horizontally, separating his head from the rest of his body—in effect, severing his neck in the picture. My faulty reasoning— conflating the wish to cause Drew harm and actually inflicting it—could easily have been pointed out by any rational adult at the time. But the fact that I may have had such a wish, and that Drew, in my mind, was now similarly "decapitated," was enough to add years of psychotherapy to anyone's life. This was the state I was in while making my first visit.

It looked like a scene from the movie *Hannibal*. As I entered Drew's room, the first thing I noticed was the Circ-O-Lectric bed that he was strapped to. In fact, it filled most of the room. It would be no exaggeration to describe the device as a cross between a torture apparatus used by a covert intelligence agency in a Third World country and something you might see as a prop in a circus for acrobatic stunts. The "bed" consisted of a pair of mammoth eight-foot-high metal rings, giant wheels, secured to a base. The rings suspended a thin mattress and sandwiching boards and sported chest, hip, and leg straps that kept Drew's almost-six-foot-tall, lean body from slipping out. The device acted sort of like a pancake flipper every two hours (24/7) to prevent skin breakdowns from developing, as he could not move his position himself or even feel the discomfort of staying in one position too long. At the head of the device were tongs with four screws drilled into Drew's skull to keep his neck from moving while the vertebrae mended.

The thing I remember most during my trip was the *drip*. At the time, Drew was positioned in his bed facing the floor, which was awkward as it was difficult to see his brown eyes when conversing. I recall he suffered from a head cold, with discharge draining from his nostrils that day. Of course, the head-down position only encouraged such drainage. It was like a slow drip from a faucet, continuous... predictable... unending. The remnants of this leakage formed a barely perceptible, slowly accumulating puddle of fluid collecting on the tiled floor below. It was a visit I could neither anticipate nor prepare for. If you were to tell me there was a young man in that room drilled to a bed with head screws and confirming the laws of gravity by watching his sinuses drain, I could not imagine.

The second thing I remember during that visit was the *itch*.

"Mitch, can you scratch my nose?"

Drew's itchy nose needed scratching, and he was in no condition to do it. *It was the first time he ever asked anything of me.* I took on the job in sort of a matter-of-fact manner, dutifully, like taking out the trash or shoveling snow. I put up a mental wall and complied. In fact, I began building walls ever since that visit. I started ignoring the smell of bodily fluids and medical paraphernalia—Betadine, latex, adhesives, bleach—that would hover under my nose in the hospital room air. I would cleanse my mind of these sick-bed distractions.

They would remain submerged from significance in my newly protected reality. The presence of incontinence or the ammonia-tinged smell of urine would hold no meaning. Later, as a physical therapist, I could immediately associate these signs with pathology; then, as a family member, I could not. It was the beginning of decades of denial.

I leaned toward Drew's head, bending my knees and hunching over. I reached forward with the hard-edged nail of my right index finger and began raking his schnoz. "Is this good?" I asked. I gently scoured it a few more times for good measure. I wondered: Scratching an itch—the littlest things that we take for granted—Drew would never do again.

The last thing I remember about the hospital stay may have been a defining moment in Drew's life, but it did not occur during my visit. My mother told me of a hospital worker, either an orderly or male nurse, who entered Drew's room to conduct some sort of medical procedure. It may have been to change a urinary catheter, clean the screws around his skull, or take blood, but whatever it was, Drew didn't want it done, at least not at that moment, and he refused. To this, the worker said something like, "Well, there is not much you can do about it, is there?" and proceeded to force the procedure upon Drew anyway, against his will. I wonder if this harrowing experience may not have had a silver lining, something that Drew may have ultimately capitalized on, drawing his attention to the rights of persons with disabilities.

The next time I saw Drew was in Manhattan, at the famous Institute for Rehabilitation Medicine, later renamed Rusk Institute. It was there that he would start his new life and first meet others like himself—people with severe disabilities.

Chapter 4. My Rehabilitation at Rusk

The institute was an interesting place to be rehabilitated. It was founded by Dr. Howard Rusk, a physician who was also one of the founders of the field of medical rehabilitation during World War II. By the time I got there, he was largely a figurehead, although he still was engaged in some of the administration of the facility. I saw him on occasion when I was a patient there, and I visited him years later, soon before his death from a stroke. A lot of people with disabilities, including myself, owe him an enormous debt of gratitude.

There is one reason that Rusk was as interesting as it was, and I assume still is: the people. Every year, a new group of patients assembled in the halls of Rusk after they had gone through their acute care, as I had. My year was certainly no exception. I am not sure whether the patients themselves would have been so intriguing if they had not been there, although they may have been; it may be that the people who found themselves at Rusk are more likely than others to be risk-takers, and risk-takers for better or worse tend to be interesting. But more than this, residing at Rusk was like being in an ongoing theatrical play, because all of us, from very different backgrounds and with very different personalities, were there for basically the same reason: to adjust to our new disabilities.

Rusk had five floors, three of which were dedicated largely to patient rooms. The first and fourth floors were for adult patients, and the fifth floor was for pediatrics. At age sixteen, I could have been sent to any of these floors, but fortunately for my sanity, I was placed in a room on the fourth floor as the youngest patient on that adult floor. Every room had four patients, and the four in my room could not have been much more different from one another.

My Roommates

One of my roommates, who was only slightly older than me, was Dave,[1] a big, African American guy who had injured himself playing a sport. He had a high-level injury like mine. Possibly, in part for this reason, and because we were close to the same age, we became good friends and often talked all night long, no doubt driving our other roommates crazy. Dave suffered from a chronically itchy nose, which is a real liability for someone with a high-level quadriplegia. Over time, he regained substantially more function than I did, though I believe he remained dependent upon the assistance of other people. Whether there is functional recovery, and the extent of it, depends very heavily upon the nature and extent of the injury and usually occurs if at all during the first year or so.

One roommate, named Ralph, was a married chemical engineer in his thirties. I can't remember how he was injured, but I remember thinking that I was glad that I was not injured at his age. His wife, who was a very nice lady, came to visit frequently, and I have every reason to believe that their marriage survived. If so, which I truly hope, it would be the exception. The marriages of a lot of the older guys fell apart, often due to nobody's fault, just that things had changed and one or the other was no longer happy. Ralph was trying to figure out how to restructure his career so that he could continue to function with limited control of his arms and no hand function. Fortunately for him, he had not only a supportive family but also a supportive employer who was willing to accommodate his disability even before it was required to do so.

In the bed next to mine was a fellow named Joe, who had gotten to this place by virtue of having attempted to dive into his family's pool from the roof of his house. If anyone is thinking of doing this, it is not advisable. He managed to break his neck upon hitting the pool floor and proceeded to come close to drowning before he was rescued. In retrospect, he probably would have been better off if he had drowned. When I met him, he already had severe bedsores all over his buttocks, and much to everyone's chagrin, he had the worst imaginable chronic diarrhea, resulting from his having swallowed a lot of chlorine. This adversely affected the ambience of our living quarters.

Joe also had the most beautiful girlfriend—a blond woman in her twenties with gigantic breasts—whom he abused every time she visited. Despite all the yelling, I always enjoyed her visits, and I thought he was out of his mind for treating her that way. I suppose he was having a rough time, which was understandable to a large extent, but I still thought that there was no excuse for verbally abusing another person, particularly a beautiful babe. She was extremely loyal but eventually broke up with him when she could not take it anymore. Later, after he was discharged from Rusk, he killed himself with an overdose of pills.

Of all the four roommates, I had the most "severe disability." I actually hate the term "severe disability," which sounds as if you have some horrible, antisocial condition; who would want to hang out with someone who was "severe"? A disability is basically just a major function limitation, no more and no less. It is true that my particular functional limitations were more substantial than anybody else's in my room and as substantial as any at Rusk at the time. This would no longer be the case, however, in that medical science is now able to save people with much more substantial disabilities, such as people who are ventilator dependent or who have major brain injuries.

The Other Players and My Theory of Rehabilitation

I have a theory explaining how medical rehabilitation works. Of course, part of it has to do with the physicians, nurses, therapists, and other dedicated health care professionals who provide services. However, I am convinced that the most important mechanism of rehabilitation occurs in the interaction of patients. In particular, I believe that one of the key components of my rehabilitation was simply looking at Joe and thinking: As screwed up as I am, thank God I am not as bad off as he is. I am sure he was thinking the same thing about me. As bad as this may sound, the knowledge that there is someone in the world more screwed up than yourself is very therapeutic.

With this in mind, let me describe just a few other members of the memorable cast of characters at Rusk that year. For example, there was a guy named Max, who returned to Rusk every once in a while with a bedsore, and who I do not believe I had ever seen without a beer can in his hand. He was a good-looking guy, probably in his late teens or early twenties, who had lower-level quadriplegia with substantial arm function and who was the boyfriend of Susan for part of the year. I was somewhat jealous of him for this, because Susan was a beautiful brunette girl who was about the same age as Max but had a lower level of injury.

Susan became a person with a disability when she was standing on a sidewalk, minding her own business, and a car went out of control, leaving the road and running into her. She could actually get around to some extent on braces and crutches, but she was in great pain all the time. Again, I was grateful that I did not have her pain, and she was no doubt grateful that she did not have my level of disability.

There was a guy across the hall named John, who was at Rusk for a long time before I got there and was there a long time afterward. He had the most severe bedsores I had ever seen and would never be able to sit up in a wheelchair for more than a couple of hours. He was a very smart guy with much more functional capacity than I had, but he was largely abandoned by his family and ultimately attempted suicide a couple of times with a knife before finally succeeding by throwing himself and his wheelchair off a roof, if the reports were correct.

It was at that time that I developed the idea that the higher one's level of injury, the higher is that individual's form of life.

There was another fellow, who lived on the first floor and was extremely good-looking. What I remember about him is that some toothpaste company hired him to be in one of their TV commercials, but they wanted him to sit on a big rock with an attractive young lady, both of them showing off their pearly white teeth. What the company did not want him to show off was his disability, which was hidden from the viewers. I found it particularly ironic that they wanted him for his physical beauty, but they apparently did not think that a person in a wheelchair could be perceived as physically beautiful.

Although I should not admit my prejudice, I did not regard this fellow as a person with a disability at all; like others with paraplegia, he had full use of his arms and hands and was fully able to take care of himself. I would always need the assistance of another person, due to my disability, which has enormous implications concerning finances, security, privacy, and a multitude of other lifestyle issues. It was at that time that I developed the idea that the higher one's level of injury, the higher is that individual's form of life. Of course, this theory was somewhat self-serving, in that it would make individuals with high-level quadriplegia, such as myself, the highest form of life. I did not hesitate to share this theory with my friends with paraplegia and low-level quadriplegia, not all of whom accepted it.

These are just a few of the cast of characters. In addition, I should mention a few of our zookeepers. My primary doctor was a rehabilitation physician named Dr. Heiner Sell, who was one of the best in the country. Tragically, he died at a relatively young age of cancer, another real loss to the field. He was replaced by his student, Dr. Kris Ragnarsson, who is another excellent physician and who is still practicing. As much as I appreciate my physicians, I always say that the nurses at Rusk were most important for my rehabilitation. The nurses were the ones who dealt with our needs on a daily basis. I fell in love with half of them that year, but I was too young for any of them to take me seriously. Still, their playful teasing made me feel like a man, and that was much appreciated as I was going through my psychological adjustment that year.

Therapists such as Pam and Gary were also very important, in that they tortured me with range-of-motion exercises that would break up the calcium adhesions that had built up in my joints when I was in the Circ-O-Lectric bed. This therapy allowed my arms to be moved in a variety of directions and was beneficial to my health as well as the flexibility needed to function well. Occupational therapists, like Toby and Sharon, with whom I also fell in love, helped develop strategies that would later help me in my education and employment.

Finally, I must mention the nurses aides, who assisted us every day with such tasks as transferring to and from our wheelchairs, dressing us, and helping us in the bathroom. One of them—nicknamed "Cupid,"[2] apparently because of all the children he had fathered, both in and out of wedlock—was a huge guy with a big heart. Another aide, named Alfred, was arguably certifiable, in that he laughed continuously, all the time. Although I did not think this was normal, I appreciated it; you cannot take yourself or your situation too seriously when your aide is laughing all the time.

The Big Debate

Although there were many interesting incidents and interactions that year, two stand out in my mind. The first was painful, and the second was kind of amusing.

The first incident resulted in the loss of the big toe on my left foot. When I was finally ready to get into a motorized wheelchair, the first chair I received was a highly sophisticated sip-and-puff chair. This was an impressive piece of technology at the time. Basically, there was a long tube from the small computer in the back of the chair, and the user would either blow into or draw air from the tube. Depending upon whether the user puffs or sips hard or soft, the chair will go forward, backward, left, or right.

I just realized that I did not mention how to stop the chair. That was actually a significant part of the problem; I was much better at starting it than stopping it. This is particularly bad when you are young and foolish, insisting upon operating the chair at full speed and refusing to place the emergency brake by your head. I believe that they are still hearing the reverberations of my collision with the elevator door at Rusk to this day. My big toe turned all different colors, got infected, and had to be amputated.

The second incident was far less traumatic but equally infuriating. The field of medical rehabilitation at that time had a classification system for assessing muscle strength, ranging from excellent (for the musculature of a limb that is not affected by paralysis) to none (for a muscle that does not operate voluntarily at all). In between, there are several intermediate categories, including good, fair, and poor, as well as pluses and minuses for each category. I had already concluded that this system was not particularly relevant to me due to the extent of my paralysis. That is, it was irrelevant, until one day one of the residents noticed a small twitch in my left biceps and proudly volunteered that he believed that it was a poor minus biceps. He was immediately interrupted by the senior physician, who indicated that this was not possible and that it was just a pulse.

So began the great biceps-pulse debate of 1973. The medical staff and some of the nursing staff started to take positions on either side—the biceps team and the pulse team. I believe that at one point it was actually a betting pool, complete with odds, in which someone could place money on either my biceps or my pulse. I remained largely neutral throughout the great debate, in that I did not really care much how it turned out, though it might have been nice to have a biceps.

The debate actually did not last long, because within a week or so it had become readily apparent that I had a tiny little biceps, which my physician immediately labeled poor minus. I was so proud! Apparently what had happened was that a tiny strand of my spinal cord must have survived my injury, and that strand allows me to flex my biceps slightly. After thirty years, it would probably be characterized now as a poor plus or maybe even a fair minus. In any event, it is really not functional, but it is fun to look at every once in a while, just as the debate was not all that important, but it was a welcome relief from the tedium of rehabilitation.

A Nice Send-off

I was at Rusk for about seven months. They were among the most important seven months I had ever spent, as well as among the most memorable. I have mentioned that my experience working with children with intellectual disabilities at the camp transformed me. Well, my injury interrupted the completion of my transformation, and my rehabilitation at Rusk completed it. I felt that I was now an adult. OK, I was a very young adult, but I felt that I was ready to take on the challenges of the world.

I feel for those people who have a disability in these days of managed care, in which people with newly developed disabilities often receive a month or so of rehabilitation, if they are lucky, or they receive care in an inappropriate facility, such as a nursing home, that is not equipped to provide intensive, comprehensive rehabilitation. Most of all, they are deprived of the luxury of adapting to their disabilities in a supportive environment in which they can interact with other similarly situated individuals, some of whom are better off, and some of whom are worse off, and most of whom are both. None of us were perfect, but we were struggling both apart and together, and we bonded that year in the knowledge that the lives we were going to live would not be easy. I think of these people often and hope they are doing well.

One of the reasons I stayed at Rusk as long as I did was that it took a while for the first floor of our house in Yonkers to become adapted to meet my needs. Nowadays, they would have thrown me out irrespective of this, and I do not know what my family would have been able to do. When I left Rusk, I was ready to leave. On my last day, which was somewhat sad, my friends threw a little party for me. They had a cake and some nice words, but the best present came at the end. Susan got up on her braces and moved slowly over to me using her crutches. Then, much to my surprise, in front of everyone, she pulled my face to hers and proceeded to stick her tongue down my throat. I had been successfully rehabilitated!

Commentary: Drew's Rehabilitation
/Mitchell Batavia, Brother/

Outside the "glottal exploratory" during Drew's send-off from Rusk, the institute was most helpful in the area of patient education. If Drew's lesion had been a bit lower, say, at cervical level C6 or 7, he would have had monumentally more functional mobility due to spared muscle activity at the elbow, and physical therapists could have trained Drew to independently get out of bed, dress himself, and push a wheelchair, with only a little help. He might have even been able to live on his own!

But this was not the case. Drew's injury was about as nosebleed high up the spine as one can climb without dying, C2-3, which meant that he would be dependent on others. It also meant that it would be in his best interests to take charge of his own care and fend off the incompetent kind. Curiously, the silver lining about his injury is that Drew never required a ventilator to breathe. In physical therapy school, you are taught that "C3-4-5 keeps the diaphragm alive." Drew's level was higher and more serious. To the extent that his injury encroached on these spinal segments in the neck, he for some miraculous reason—perhaps due to fiber sparing—escaped the consequences of this sobering mnemonic.[3] He could breathe on his own!

The institute did teach Drew the importance of taking care of himself: to avoid bedsores, evade pneumonia, and dodge bladder infections, all occupational hazards of having a spinal cord injury. In fact, if you were to visit Drew's home at any time during his life, you would never see him far from a large container of microwaved tea with a protruding catheter-size straw that he would intermittently sip from between bouts of typing or debating, in an attempt to bathe his kidneys, flush his bladder, and stave off a dreaded urinary tract infection. Now, I know what you may be thinking: "Urinary tract infection? What's the big deal? Take a course of Amoxicillin for seven to fourteen days, and you're back on your feet." But the risk of infection is quite high with Drew's condition. Bacteria can colonize and take up residence along the lining of a bladder that does not empty fully. And Drew's bladder likely did not empty fully, possibly contributing to these ongoing infections.[4]

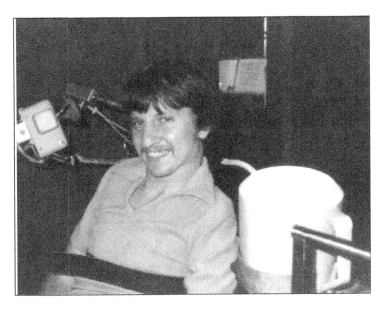

Drew always had a pot of tea nearby to keep him hydrated.

Drew had low-grade urinary tract infections during much of his postaccident life, punctuated by more serious ones, for which he repeatedly took antibiotics. And antibiotic overuse, as we now know, can lead to the development of drug-resistant strains of bacteria. If these bug strains get into the bloodstream, they can spread like wildfire throughout the body, causing massive inflammation. Vital organs then begin to shut down. To make matters worse, urinary tract infections are not always reliably detected in persons with spinal cord injuries. In Drew's case, profuse sweating and unrelenting muscle spasms hinted that something was brewing. Drinking fluids was one key to prevention at the time. And one of the few perks of being a patient with a spinal cord injury, as I recall, was a "beer prescription." Drew boasted that drinking beer, with its pee-promoting, diuretic qualities, helped flush his bladder. I doubt this was an official medical recommendation.

The institute also offered Drew a pair of legs. He needed legs to get to clinic, to get to classes, and to get on with his life. For people with quadriplegia, these new legs came in the guise of a power (a.k.a. motorized or electric) wheelchair, an extension of his body that allowed him not only to saunter but to run. You have likely seen these magnificent machines sprinting down streets. They typically sport metal tubing, padded armrests, and draped seat upholstery, often topped with a racecar-style bucket seat. Two pairs of wheels spin, smaller ones in the front to change direction when one's mind changes, and larger ones in the rear, powered by a car battery. To steer this jewel, a person possessing chin movements need only use a rubberized chin toggle and direct one's chin upward to go forward, downward to go backward, left to go...well, you get it. Initially, Drew used a sip-and-puff control mechanism (using breath) to operate his chair, but eventually he resorted to chin control.

Power wheelchairs revolutionized independent mobility for people like Drew. And the best thing about them is that once Drew was placed in his chair, he was independent for much of his day. No longer would he be pushed around by others; instead, he could plot his own route and chart his own destiny, and he could do so solo—unless, of course, it broke down.

And the first problem with power chairs is that they break down, fairly regularly, in fact. When Drew's power chair lost its charge around midnight in Georgetown and Cheryl had to push the chair home, they arrived at their doorstop at two in the morning. On another occasion, the chair just started up on its own and almost propelled Drew through his eighth-floor apartment window in Southwest Washington, DC. In retrospect, aberrant behavior like this is not uncommon with assisted technology.

However, the feature I most want to emphasize is the chair's weight—it's army-tank heavy. So if the wheelchair breaks down, someone else needs to push this "small car," placed in neutral, from behind. It's sort of like pushing a 450-pound paperweight.

Below are two family accounts of wheelchair woes. The first is from our mother, Renée, who discovered the hillside beauty of Berkeley's 1,200-acre campus.

Upon his arrival at the University of California, Berkeley, Drew made arrangements to visit a local health facility to hook up with a doctor and familiarize him with his condition. Drew and I were transported there by a school van. The visit proved to be longer than planned, and the van that had dropped us off never returned to pick us up. In order to return to the dorms, I pushed him in his heavy electric chair, which could not navigate the hilly terrain, for two miles uphill.

The second account is from Cheryl, who found similar challenges with Drew's wheelchair on a footbridge in Florida.

There was (and hopefully still is) a picturesque, steeply arched, narrow, white-stuccoed, and probably historic-landmarked footbridge over a canal in Miami Beach. The apex of that lovely bridge is an absolutely terrible place for a motorized wheelchair to break down. Let me assure you that there are many such steep, isolated, uncomfortable places to get stuck in a motorized wheelchair. Drew located his share of them in patched-up chairs that he had literally run to death, using them as his primary means of transportation. He expended a tremendous amount of his valuable time and energy on repairs and on trying to get approval for replacement.

Another problem with power wheelchairs is cost. This may be a good time to warn you that if you ever did toy with the idea of becoming a person with a severe physical disability, please do factor in these costs. There are the requisite home renovations for accessibility, the high-roofed adapted van, the paid attendant, the medical expenses (more on this later), and, of course, the wheelchair. The chair is not unlike a Cadillac purchase, especially when you tack on all the bells and whistles: power tilt, high-end skin-protective cushions, and programmable cruise control.

But the reason I bring up cost is that after a slew of breakdowns in an aging chair, Drew would try to obtain a new one. This is expected about every five years, when the usefulness of this equipment maxes out. Getting it paid for, however, is another story. Insurance companies typically resisted this temptation, although profits would never be mentioned in their denial letters.

In an article titled, "Of Wheelchairs and Managed Care" in the journal *Health Affairs*, Drew describes a surreal exchange with his physician's office manager and gatekeeper, Ms. Johnson, who would not support a prescription for a new wheelchair, because his existing one could likely continue to be repaired, perhaps indefinitely.[5]

Me: I am very disturbed that Dr. Harris will not write a prescription for my new chair, Ms. Johnson. My current chair is falling apart.

Ms. Johnson: I spoke with a representative from your PPO, who informed me that they are willing to pay for the repair of your chair but not for a new one.

Me: But each time it needs to be repaired I won't have the use of it. My wheelchair-repair person has informed me that my current chair is at the end of its useful life and breakdowns are likely to become more and more frequent. Every time it breaks down, the effect on me is similar to as if your legs just stopped working. I can't work, I can't pick up my kids from school, and it could be hazardous if the chair breaks down in the middle of a street.

Ms. Johnson: I am just telling you what your company told me.

Me: Okay, if that's the case, why don't you just give me the prescription and I'll fight it out with the PPO.

Ms. Johnson: The doctor won't write the prescription for you.

Me: Why not?

Ms. Johnson: How are we to know if you really need a new chair or if the current chair can still be fixed? If we were to write the prescription, and you do not really need a new chair, we could be subject to claims of health care fraud.

Me: I teach health care law. It's extremely unlikely that you would be subject to such claims if you indicate in good faith that I am a quadriplegic with a wheelchair that is over five years old and in growing disrepair.

Ms. Johnson: We do not know if the chair can still be fixed.

Me: Any piece of equipment can still be fixed. The question is whether it's worthwhile doing so. Your car could be fixed indefinitely, but you probably wouldn't want to have to rely on it if it were in the repair shop half of the time. How would you get to work? I have the same problem with my wheelchair.

Ms. Johnson: Do you know how much this new wheelchair will cost? About $24,000. We all end up paying for that. The company has a right to decide whether a new chair is needed or whether the current chair can be repaired.

Me: First, I know how much the chair will cost. It is a highly customized, sophisticated piece of equipment. Do you think I am happy about its price? I'll have to pay about 20 percent of that cost in deductibles and copayments. That's a substantial amount of money out of pocket, and I can assure you that I would not order this chair unless I absolutely needed it. Second, you are right that it is for the company to decide, not you. Now, will you ask Dr. Harris to write the prescription?

Ms. Johnson: No, I won't. You can have your current chair repaired.

Me: Why do you think you know so much about my chair? How do you know that my chair can still be repaired productively?

Ms. Johnson: My grandmother is in a similar chair.

Me: Your grandmother must be a high-level quadriplegic. How unusual! There are only a few customized chairs like mine in the country, and she has one of them.

The decibel level of this discourse rose as the discussion grew more and more bizarre. Toward the end it became clear that this doctor's office would not resolve the dilemma.

See full article here:
http://content.healthaffairs.org/content/18/6/177.full.pdf+html

One Other Benefit of Rusk
/Mitchell Batavia, Brother/

There was one additional benefit of Rusk, but it was mine. During Drew's recovery, I floundered about choosing careers. Having been at Rusk, Drew knew of a summer health program where young men and women were exposed to health care careers. I applied in 1978 and was accepted as a Reader's Digest Fellow. We were nicknamed "yellow jackets" because of the coats we wore. It was a good experience, in that I discovered a talent. One day I caught a patient from falling in the gym before physical therapists could get to him. It was something I seemed to be good at, and we all want to be good at something. I saw the marriage of biology and personal manual service to others as a good fit. I went to physical therapy school and landed my first job at, of all places, Rusk.

Like many health care providers, I suppose, I was propelled into this field by family tragedy. Perhaps there's a psychological need to fix your family. But any notion that I could, through professional training, help Drew recover from his spinal injury would prove delusional and was something I would struggle with for years. And the reality is that no one could help Drew, and *he never wanted it*. At the time, spinal cord regeneration was just not a serious conversation in medical circles; the scarring of the injury site interfered with reinnervation—the reconnecting process of nerves—and even now the cure is not "just around the corner," as Drew's physicians first told him. As reality was utterly bleak, I even fancied bizarre "what-if" cures as a distraction, like suppose the answer to spinal cord regeneration turned out to be as sublimely simple as scrubbing the scar-ridden neural tract endings with an abrasive cleaner, toothpaste perhaps, with fluoride an added bonus. If only reality was that ludicrous. It's times like those when your best bet just may be praying to a higher authority.

Chapter 5. Definitive Proof of God

I have little use for organized religion, which just has too many rules for my taste. However, this does not mean that I do not believe in God. In fact, I have a very deep belief in an almighty creative force, which I call God. My belief in God has not come easily. For some people, the existence of a life force itself is adequate evidence of the existence of God. It is not that I am not in awe of the life force, as evidenced by the frenetic energy and intelligence of my children and even my dog, Clifford. This is truly remarkable and clearly offers evidence of God. The fact that I survived my substantial injuries to live a good life is further evidence. However, this was still not enough. I needed a miracle providing definitive proof of God. I got my miracle toward the end of my stay at Rusk.

Looking for God at Rusk

The year of my rehabilitation was not an easy year. I was in almost constant discomfort. For the first year after my injury, every time I would get up in my wheelchair, I would be dizzy for several hours. Individuals with quadriplegia tend to have very low blood pressure, and particularly after being bedridden for several months, it took a long time for my body to adjust to sitting up. Moreover, my body was adjusting to other physiologic changes as well.

In particular, due to the loss of the ability to voluntarily control my bladder, my entire urinary tract system was adjusting to my need to empty my bladder automatically. As a result, I perspired virtually nonstop that year. On an average day, I would go through three or four shirts, from which pools of sweat could be wrung out. This was uncomfortable generally, but even more so during the winter, when the halls of the hospital were sometimes cold. I spent a lot of time that year just wondering whether these problems would ever subside so that I could live a relatively comfortable life.

Even more challenging and difficult than the physiologic adjustment was the initial psychological adjustment. People often ask me how long it took for me to accept my disability. Many do not believe me when I say that I accepted it, for the most part, within a few months. This is not to say that I did not have occasional periods of minor depression during the first two years, but these were not severe, and virtually all teenagers have occasional fits of depression.

I believe that there was an interesting mechanism by which I adjusted to my disability. First, I was in a lot of pain from my car accident. Then, once the initial pain had subsided, I started perspiring profusely. Over time, the sweating subsided. At each stage, I was simply so happy to be relieved of the pain and discomfort that the disability did not seem like such a big deal. I was also very relieved that I had already experienced many of the physical experiences I wanted to have before becoming disabled.

Psychic Pain

So why was I having a difficult time psychologically? I was very worried that year. I was worried that my injury would destroy my family. I could never let them know how uncomfortable I was, because I was concerned that they would fall apart. I was particularly concerned for my father, who would have traded places with me in a minute. He does not handle my suffering very well, and consequently I did not share it with him. As much as I was concerned about him and my other family members, I was at least equally concerned that my injury and all the expenses associated with it would break my family financially. I had received a relatively small settlement from the insurance company of the driver responsible for my injury, and this was, fortunately, enough to cover my medical expenses. However, it was not nearly enough to finance the enormous expenses that were still to come.

My physical problems and my financial anxiety both related to yet another concern: getting through eleventh grade that year. As I mentioned already, my injury took place in the summer after my sophomore year. I had an extremely strong academic record until this time, and I was committed to maintaining that record and graduating with the same high school class with which I started high school. There was just one problem with this plan. I spent the first three months of the academic year in a Circ-O-Lectric bed, in which it was not so easy to study.

New York State did send a teacher to my hospital room every once in a while, but that individual usually arrived inebriated, and in any event, I was in no shape to engage in any serious studying. This situation did not get much better after I arrived at Rusk, which had a one-room schoolhouse on the fifth floor in which one elderly teacher attempted to teach virtually every subject. Again, with all the perspiring and other problems, I was not in any condition to study.

My Miracle: Divine Intervention

To make things worse, in New York State the most challenging year academically is eleventh grade. That is the year that each student must take four Regents examinations, which are very challenging statewide comprehensive tests of knowledge, each of which addresses a specific subject. In ninth grade, there was one Regents examination, and in tenth grade there were two. I had done very well on these. However, in eleventh grade, I was to take exams in chemistry, trigonometry, English, and history. Unfortunately, I knew nothing about the first two subjects and almost nothing about the New York State curriculum for the second two subjects. Consequently, for the first time in my life, I was going to fail everything. This would ruin all of the plans I had for many years, including plans to graduate with my class and to get into a good college.

If I was sweating for most of that year as a result of my injury, I was really sweating during the months of May and June, trying to catch up on a year's worth of work in a couple of months without the benefit of a teacher who knew the subject matter. Things were not looking at all good. My cumulative grade point average for my entire high school career was about to do a nosedive, which would have ruined my prospects for getting into a good school. I was distraught, but I kept studying despite all the pain and discomfort, hoping that I could pull it all together at the last minute. In retrospect, I realize, this would have been impossible under the circumstances.

It was just a couple of days before the exam, and I was really anxious about it. I turned the TV on, and the news commentator made the most remarkable announcement: "For the first time ever, the Regents examinations have been canceled this year." I stared at the TV incredulously. I figured that all of the last-minute cramming had made me delusional and that I was hearing things that I wanted to hear. However, the announcer went on talking about how the Regents exams were stolen that year, and that there was not enough time for officials to develop new exams. The best part, at least from my perspective, was that the exams apparently were stolen by yeshiva students. These are Jewish students in religious academies who traditionally have been known for their academic excellence and high ethical standards.

Now, I know that some of you may be thinking that this situation really does not rise to the level of a miracle. If so, I would like to know your standards for a miracle. This was the first time in my entire life that I was not prepared academically for anything, and it is the first time the Regents examinations were ever canceled. Moreover, the exams were canceled because people of my own ethnicity had stolen them. This is all too much of a coincidence for me, and I believe some people have been elevated to sainthood by achieving miracles that were no more impressive. If this was not divine intervention, I do not know what is!

Chapter 6. You Can Go Home Again, at Least for a Year

I am generally not a very lucky person. I am one of those people who chooses "heads" and it comes up "tails," and vice versa, ninety-nine times out of a hundred. The fact that I was the only one in my high school to manage to fly through a windshield and break his neck the first time he ever hitchhiked is some indication of my luck. Being generally unlucky is a good thing, because you learn very early not to be a gambler; when you gamble, you always lose. This does not mean that I do not take risks. I take risks all the time, but they are carefully calculated risks with very good odds, because I know that if the odds are even or worse, I will always lose.

Yet in some ways, and in some of the most important ways, I have been very lucky. I have already said that I was extremely lucky in being born to my family. If you have to be a generally unlucky person, it is good when the few occasions in which you are lucky have the most important consequences. As I indicated in the previous chapter, I was either extraordinarily lucky that I did not fail the eleventh grade or, as I prefer to believe, God intervened directly on my behalf. I recognize that this interpretation could reflect some mental defect on my part, but I believe that having some delusions of grandeur can be extremely helpful in surviving in this world, hence the idea that God would personally intervene on my behalf.

I also got lucky when I returned to my neighborhood in Yonkers after my rehabilitation. My house was built in a way that allowed my parents to modify the first floor so that we could set up my bedroom there. Many other people lived in houses or apartments that could not be adapted, and many others did not have the resources to do such a modification. Money is extremely important in being able to get the services and equipment needed by people with disabilities, and most of these individuals have very little money. Even those in the middle class, such as my family, are challenged by all the enormous costs of living with a disability, including purchasing an accessible van and modifying a house.

Almost as important as the accessibility of my home was the accessibility of my school. Lincoln High School, where I completed my freshman and sophomore years, was only one long block from our house, and I used to walk to school all the time. I really would not have wanted to start a new school in my senior year. Luckily, or with divine intervention, Lincoln High School was the only school in Yonkers at the time that was fully accessible to people using wheelchairs. I would be able to return to my old school and my old friends.

You Can Go Home Again

I mentioned that I was fortunate that, in those days, people with injuries could stay in rehabilitation for a substantial period of time. All together, between my acute care and rehabilitation, I was away from home for about nine months. The negative side of this is that when you are in health care institutions for an extended period of time, you develop a kind of institutional mentality. This is not to say that you enjoy living in such institutions; even the best of them, such as Rusk, require you to conform to their schedule.

Most institutions are very impersonal places, and while this was not true of Rusk, with all its wonderful people, Rusk was not like home. Yet this institutional mentality you develop gives you a sense of security that is very comforting when you have it, and initially disconcerting when you do not. Even though you do not necessarily enjoy the inconveniences and lack of privacy of being there, you know that all of your needs will eventually be addressed. Much like a drug, the longer that you are addicted to this sense of security, which is not always even real security, the harder it is to free yourself from it. I had been in rehabilitation for a fairly long time, and consequently the transition to living at home was somewhat challenging.

Of course, the shock of this transition was also absorbed by the support of my wonderful family. I simply do not know how I would have made it without them, and I truly feel for those people with disabilities who do not have the support of strong families. I believe that this is the single most important factor determining whether a person with a disability succeeds in this world. Again, I really lucked out in this essential regard.

My First Personal Assistants

In addition to adapting our house, my parents had placed an advertisement in the newspaper and hired a fellow originally from the island of Grenada to serve as my personal assistant. This may require a little explanation. A lot of people think that if you have a major disability, you require the assistance of health care professionals for the rest of your life. It is, of course, true that people with disabilities, like other people, require the assistance of health care professionals when we become ill. It is also true that many people with disabilities, particularly older people, rely upon health care professionals to satisfy their long-term care and personal assistance needs. They do so by living either in nursing homes or other institutions that provide care, or at home, with home health aides typically provided by home health agencies.

However, it is not true that people with disabilities have to receive their care and assistance through health care professionals. A large and growing number of people with disabilities receive such services from people who are not trained as health care professionals, under what has been referred to as the independent living model of long-term care. I recently published a book on this model. The independent living model has served as the basis for my care for the past thirty years, as well as that of many of my friends. Because it does not rely upon health care professionals, it tends to be much more affordable than the medical model, and many people with disabilities, including myself, strongly prefer to train our own personal assistants to meet our needs the way we want them to be met. Under the independent living model, the person with a disability is the boss, and I have been an employer of personal assistants for a very long time.

Ivan was the very first of my personal assistants. My parents, whose only previous experience in such matters was hiring a few housekeepers over the years (which is really a very similar process), did a good job in hiring him. He was responsible, diligent, and a good guy, and we had some good times together. He lived with us during the week and went to his home in Brooklyn during the weekends, on his days off. On occasion, he would take me to his neighborhood, where I was typically the only white person to be found. I always enjoyed those visits, and everyone treated me very well.

Ivan stayed with us for much of my first year at home after rehabilitation. Eventually, he decided to move on, and we had to hire a new assistant. This time, my parents did not do as well. I actually cannot remember this fellow's name, which may be because I have consciously blocked it from my memory. It was not that this guy, who was also from the Caribbean, was a bad guy. He did his best, but he was no Ivan. A lot of the problem was that he had almost no short-term memory, a condition that he may well have developed as a result of long-term use of a variety of drugs.

Every morning, I would have to teach this fellow all over again the routine of getting me dressed and into my wheelchair. Although this got rather old after a while, it gave me excellent experience in training a new assistant, which I did basically every day he worked for us. The other lesson I learned from this experience was that I was going to have to start hiring my assistants myself. As much as my parents did their best in the hiring process, I would have to bear the consequences of the hiring decision, and I would have to get very good at this.

For better or worse, this fellow stayed with me through the end of my senior year and through the first week of college.

Back to School

I returned to Lincoln High School in September and was greeted almost like a wounded war hero, although having a car accident is admittedly less worthy of admiration than becoming disabled in battle. The timing for my return was very good. I had gone home from Rusk in June, and therefore I had the entire summer to adjust to being back in my neighborhood. During the summer, a lot of old friends and some new ones dropped by to see how I was doing. Some of them had visited me in rehabilitation, and I really appreciated that. I did my very best to make them feel comfortable with my disability, a skill that I have since perfected to the extent that many people say they forget that I have a disability after being with me for a little while.

Some of my old friends I did not see much that year. This included some of the guys who used to play sports with me and who were having a lot of difficulty in dealing with my new situation. I never held this against them, and I still regard them as good friends. I can remember, back when I was running long-distance, that one day during a run I encountered a man in a wheelchair, and just seeing him gave me such psychological discomfort that it made me run with a pronounced limp. If I was so uncomfortable in dealing with the disability of a total stranger prior to my injury, how could I not understand the discomfort of my friends, who just a few months earlier were playing basketball with me?

One person I did not see as much as I would have liked that year was Lisa. It is not that she did not drop by, which she did every once in a while, but every time we were together, there was so much pain in her eyes that I did not encourage her to stick around. She was going through her own personal issues, and dealing with mine at the same time was too much. Years later, she told me how my injury devastated her.

One time, during the summer, Lisa dropped by my house, and we went off on our own and kissed for a long time. This was wonderful on the one hand and extraordinarily painful on the other. I did not see much of Lisa during our senior year. It was just too painful for her, and I understood. Even though she was not with me physically, I felt her support with me all the time that year and ever since. As a grown woman with a family in New York, who, remarkably, became a surgical nurse notwithstanding her early aversion to dissecting frogs, she remains one of my dearest friends.

I met many other new friends my senior year who had not known me before my injury. This gave me a sense of how people would respond to me when I would go to college the next year. Large numbers of students were attracted to me for some reason, and I was almost always surrounded by people. My mother's greatest fear, that I would end up being lonely (a fear that I never really had), did not seem as if it was going to be much of a problem.

My Early Political Career

In the beginning of our senior year, there was an election for class officers. For some reason that I do not fully understand to this day, I decided to run for senior class president. Of course, the responsibilities of senior class officers were extremely limited, and this was mostly a figurehead position. I suppose running for class office was my way of jumping back into life. My opponent that year was a fellow named George, who was a friend and a popular guy in the class. To be absolutely honest, I do not know who won the election. I know that I got a substantial number of votes, but I honestly do not know whether I got as many as George did. Maybe I did, but it would have been quite a coincidence if the election was actually a tie, which is what we were told.

One of the worst things about having a disability is that you often do not know for certain whether your achievements are based strictly on merit or whether someone is just trying to protect you from pain. (It should be noted that people with disabilities are not by any means the only ones who have this problem; for example, people from wealthy and influential families also have it.) As I have already said, I do not want to be protected and would have preferred to be told that I lost, if in fact I had. I will probably never know. In any event, George and I served as copresidents of the senior class of Lincoln High School in the school year of 1974-75, and that worked out just fine.

Prom Night

The senior class officers actually did have one important responsibility that year: to plan the senior prom. I was very involved in this planning, and I attended the dinner at the restaurant where, we all agreed, it would be held. Ironically, while I would help to plan the event, I would not personally attend the senior prom. I just did not feel up to it that soon after my injury. I would have had to ask some young lady to join me, and I was concerned that she would feel compelled to say yes. Even if she did say yes, I would have had to deal with the realities that I would have to be fed by her and that I did not dance very well (not that I danced very well before my injury).

Clearly, I still needed to work through some of these issues in my own mind before I started engaging in social affairs. On the evening of the prom, I was very happy to be home with my family, and I had no remorse or regrets at all. I was pleased to learn the following day that everyone had a good time. If things had gone very differently the previous year, Lisa would have been my date that evening (assuming that she had said yes), but that was not meant to be.

Overall, our senior year was enjoyable, but not terribly interesting or exciting. We were just basically spending time, waiting to begin the next stages of our lives. Probably the most exciting incident for me that year was when my wheelchair did not respond to my command to stop and proceeded to move toward the giant glass window in the front hall of the school, running out of energy just a few feet before

I would have crashed through it. As much as I wanted an exciting life, I could have done without such excitement.

On another occasion, one of my wheels stopped working, causing my chair to go in circles for what seemed to be a very long time, until one of my fellow students was able to stop it. I imagine that this looked fairly ridiculous to anyone who was in the hallway at the time, with the exception of those innocent bystanders who were too busy attempting to dodge my chair before it mowed them down. Such situations taught me an important lesson early: When these things happen, the best way to deal with them is to simply laugh at yourself. The worst thing you can do is take yourself or the situation too seriously.

Getting Ready for College

Most of our senior year was dedicated to preparing for the rest of our lives. For about half of the class, this meant applying to several colleges of their choice. I ultimately graduated twenty-first in my class of a little over 500 students, putting me in the top 5 percent. Those of us in that group were mostly applying to some of the top schools in the country, including Ivy League schools like Harvard, Yale, and Princeton. Deciding where to apply was very confusing to many of my fellow high achievers. The decision was much simpler for me.

I was told that there were basically three schools in the country that could accommodate my needs: the University of California, Berkeley; the University of Illinois; and the University of California, Riverside. This decision was what would later be called a "no-brainer." Nobody had ever heard of UC Riverside. The University of Illinois, which established one of the first programs for students with disabilities in the country, seemed like it would be uninhabitable for about seven months of the year. Fortunately, UC Berkeley was arguably the top public university in the country, with as many Nobel Prize winners as the Ivy League schools.

I applied to UC Berkeley and was accepted. I was going to Berkeley or, as some people called it, Bezerkeley.

Commentary: The Return to Yonkers
/Mitchell Batavia, Brother/

When Drew returned home from Rusk, the ground floor of our Crawford Street home had been revamped to welcome a wheelchair. Our den was converted into a bedroom and housed a queen-size waterbed to keep bedsores at bay. Our eating nook was transformed into a roll-in shower room, and our kitchen counter was replaced with an elevated one, high enough to clear Drew's knees so he could roll his wheelchair under it to eat with the rest of the family. Lastly, a concrete ramp was built against the brick outer wall of our garage, allowing Drew to roll into the house through our kitchen door. Wheelchair friendly was our home, and Drew was its focal point.

You may wonder whether our family dynamics shifted with this new focal point. Drew was the firstborn, and I would be hard pressed to say that birth order never had an impact; libraries of textbooks argue otherwise. But following his accident, it was tacitly understood that he and his needs came first, and everyone else—including my sister, Donna, and I—had to eke out a late childhood with what remained. All energy, attention, and protection went his way.

I'm not sure to what extent Donna was affected by Drew's return. She was of independent mind and had a decent social life and support system outside the home. And I finally had a bedroom that I did not have to share with anyone—a creepy, positive side-effect of this family tragedy. Oddly, I did not feel the negative effects of Drew's return. Having been left to my own devices growing up probably prepared me well for Drew's homecoming, when my parents, but particularly my mother, had to triage and tend almost exclusively to his care, an experience I wish on no parent, and what must have been a soul-crushing existence.

My mother insists our new family configuration did impact Donna and me. Our lives certainly circled around Drew, and perhaps it provided a sense of purpose in some mildly disturbing way: getting Drew out of bed, positioning him in his wheelchair, handling bouts of dizziness, managing episodes of choking, locking the wheelchair safely in the van, practicing deep-breathing exercises. Helping with these tasks provided a feeling of competence, as if one could be entrusted with special knowledge. One day, Drew even trained me to apply his external latex urinary catheter (perhaps his attendant was unavailable). Uncomfortable recollections like these sink and resurface as family roles became blurred but never outwardly questioned. Was I an adolescent or an adult, sibling or assistant, son or servant? It mattered not. Tribal obligation extinguished these unacceptable thoughts; you do it because you are family, because you care, because it needs to get done. And done it gets. Even so, ambivalence lingers when helping roles are acquired through mandate. But life went on, and so did the Batavia family.

The Poems

It was during that year that Drew began writing poetry, largely to kill boredom and likely to give expression. He had great talent and was prolific during that senior year of high school, writing well over twenty pieces, perhaps even forty, a yield that hinted at his future success in publishing.

"At My Window" touches on the wish for independence, a concept that he would write about later in his life as part of the independent living movement. His opening verse:

> As I sit by my bedroom window
> Gazing out at the world so free
> Window seems like the bars of a prison.
> My greatest wish is to find the key

Drew hints at his future mission and the work that he will need to achieve in the following verse from "Rolling Slowly."

> My tread marks shout out "I was here"
> Or are they crying "rest, be near,"
> But so far away are my goals
> And so, my tired wheelchair rolls

"Individuality," a poem he dedicated to our cousin, Neil Marcus, may have also reflected Drew's continual need to learn and develop a unique and highly sought after skill set, which he amassed through diverse college and employment experiences in government and the private sector over his lifetime.

> He's a wanderer to complete his quest
> All over the land with an occasional rest
> Takes temporary jobs
> To keep sheltered and dressed,
> For dependence is one thing
> He'll always detest.

And in the first and last verses of "Not Accessible to All," Drew more than hints at his mission of a barrier-free world, foreshadowing his future involvement in the Americans with Disabilities Act of 1990.

"NOT ACCESSIBLE TO ALL"
The sign upon the subway wall
By stairs that I can't climb
The prejudices of the time
Inscribed in letters very bold,
Cold and old and growing mold,
Premonition of a fall

Rise up. The sign has been attacked
Join freedom's underground railroad,
A million who for years have lacked
Will rise up and demand what's owed.
Rise up! Your weakness is your strength
A thousand times you've paid the toll.
Rise up! We've been held back too long.
It's time that wheels must roll.

But Drew's favorite poem, and mine too, was "The Tree of Blue" a poem about how limited adult thinking can destroy a child's dream by advising on how things ought to be rather than how they can be.

He gazed the world
And what he saw,
The child, so young,
Began to draw.

What great wonders
Came to his eyes
His crayons drew
Bright yellow skies.

A big green dog
Lay on his bed
The uncut grass
(Its color red).

But what stood out
In the child's view,
Last, he sketched
The tree of blue.

Then a man saw
This paradise;
He said that it
Was very nice.

"But I'm afraid
It isn't right,
An illusion of
Your untrained sight

For grass is green,
The sky is blue,
And the tree played
A trick on you."

So just like those
In this man's youth
Who taught him
Reality's truth

He too passed
The curse along
And told the child
That he was wrong

And this is how
A man can blind
The world's beauty
From a child's mind.

And how they both
Now wish to see
The beautiful
Blue tree.

Drew submitted his poems to a publisher, and predictably the feedback, although gentle, was annoying: the poems rhymed. Drew's "tree" was clearly too blue for him. Fortunately, Drew, the optimist, never recycled these limited worldviews on others, and certainly not on himself. Otherwise, how would he have accomplished what he did in his lifetime?

The Art

Also around this time, Drew asked me to create art for him. Back then, I was (along with others) under the illusion that I had some natural talent for the craft. In truth, I could draw a bit better than straight lines and color between them. I didn't know at the time that his request for art held any particular significance; it did.

The art, a plaque with Friedrich Nietzsche's aphorism, "What does not kill me makes me stronger," was a two-line wood etching. I carved the letters with a chisel and then burned the wood edges to give the panel the appearance of having been created by a higher power, sort of like the Ten Commandments. I started to run out of space toward the end of the second line at "stronger," squishing the letters together to keep the whole phrase on the panel, but, as I said, my talent was likely not in art. With regard to the quote, Nietzsche may have actually said, "What makes *us* stronger" or perhaps "makes *you* stronger," but no matter. If a situation didn't kill you, you probably became smarter, better, stronger, tougher, quicker, or wiser for it. Drew lived by this quote. He was subjected to a never-ending series of life hurdles and torments, and yet surmounted and became more resilient after each one.

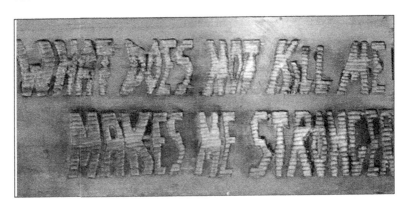

The wooden plaque with Friedrich Nietzsche's aphorism, "What does not kill me makes me stronger," commissioned by Drew and carved by his brother, Mitchell.

Drew also requested a second piece of art, an adaptation of a Pablo Picasso drawing, *Don Quixote,* which depicts a knight on a horse facing windmills, which I recreated with pen and ink. But Drew wanted Don Quixote *mounted in a wheelchair* rather than on a horse, sporting a spear and facing his mortal enemy, the windmills of injustice. Drew viewed these windmills not as imaginary threats but as real ones that infringed on civil rights, the rights of those with disabilities. Throughout Drew's lifetime, this knockoff print hung on his office wall, serving as a reminder of a mission he would later adopt. But to fulfill this mission, Drew would first need to go to college.

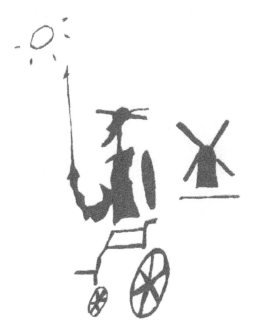

Don Quixote mounted on a wheelchair
and fighting the windmills of injustice

Chapter 7. Go West, Young Man, to Bezerkeley

In the 1960s and early 1970s, Berkeley, California, had to be one of the most interesting places to live in the United States. This was the center of many of the nationally publicized campus protests on a variety of issues ranging from opposition to the Vietnam War to civil rights to environmental issues. If there was an issue to protest, Berkeley was the place for it. I arrived at Berkeley in late August 1975, which was the very end of this great era of civil protests. I lived for that year in Cunningham Hall, a large dormitory just a block or so away from the famous People's Park, a relatively small green area that served as the site for many of the protests.

I have been told recently that Berkeley, or at least the UC Berkeley campus, has become very conservative and boring in current times, though this is difficult to believe. Even when I was there, which was well after the major turmoil, Berkeley was anything but conservative or boring. I do not know when Berkeley was first characterized as Bezerkeley, but it was a result of the predominant hippie culture that prevailed at the time. One could hardly imagine an environment that was less conducive to academic study, particularly for a young man on his own for the first time.

Getting to Berkeley

When most people go off to college, it entails a substantial transition, including the need to transport a lot of stuff to campus. For a person with a disability such as mine, the task is exponentially more difficult. Part of this is simply because we require and have more stuff. This includes wheelchairs, wheelchair cushions, other durable medical equipment, and tons of supplies. However, this still is not, by any means, the most significant aspect of the transition. People with disabilities develop support systems within their communities to assist them in dealing with the challenges of independent living, such as transportation systems, durable medical equipment suppliers, health care providers, and personal assistants.

My mother and Grandpa Joe accompanied me on the plane trip to San Francisco, which is across the bay from Berkeley. My mom is not a big drinker; she would occasionally have a drink or two at a social occasion, but never more than that. I never saw my mother drink so much as when we were on that jet. This unusual behavior no doubt reflected her anxiety over the prospect of leaving her first son, who had no use of his arms, legs, and hands, in one of the strangest places in the entire world. The extent of its strangeness became immediately apparent. I will never forget my grandfather's double take when he entered the unisex bathroom in my dormitory hall and was greeted by my soon-to-be friend, Bonnie, in her underwear, with toothpaste all over her mouth and shaving cream on her legs.

My mother's anxiety proved justifiable in a very short period of time. My first official act in Berkeley was to run my wheelchair off a curb and into the street. The piddling little six-volt wheelchair that I had received in New York was simply not up to handling the substantial hills of Berkeley.

Therefore, the first order of business was to order a new twenty-four-volt motorized wheelchair. Unfortunately, I would not receive the new chair until close to the end of the first semester. This presented a significant transportation problem.

I resolved this problem by taking up hitchhiking again; this time, rather than hitchhiking in cars, which I have learned can be hazardous to your health, I waved over any student who looked like he or she was going in my direction to push me to my destination. Remarkably, this was how I got places, including my classes, in my first few months at Berkeley. Whatever shyness I might have had before this experience was lost by the time I received my new wheelchair.

Unfortunately, my mother and grandfather became well aware of this transportation problem, which did not do much for their anxiety level. I learned, at an early stage of this experience, not to share any of my crises with my family, because all it would do is increase anxiety without resolving the issue. Of course, this was not an option this time, because my family was with me. To make things worse, I developed a bad bladder infection during my first week at Berkeley, and I had to go to a doctor.

Fortunately, the Center for Independent Living in Berkeley, the first independent living center to assist people with disabilities living in the community, had an accessible van service for such emergencies. They took me, with my mother and grandfather, to the doctor's office in the late afternoon one day. Unfortunately, they forgot to pick us up after the appointment. Consequently, my mother, who was not a young woman at the time, had to push me the two or three miles back to the dormitory. She and I were not impressed.

This raises an important issue concerning services for people with disabilities at Berkeley at the time. When I applied to the university, my family made numerous inquiries concerning the services that would be available to me. University officials certainly talked a very good game. They conveyed the impression that the organizations responsible for providing the services I needed had been around for a very long time. Actually, this was not exactly true. The Center for Independent Living had been established about two years earlier. Although it was true that the residential program for students with disabilities had been established several years earlier, it was initially at Cowell Hospital on campus, and it had only recently moved to the dormitories, which was an entirely different animal.

Irrespective of the marketing, the Berkeley infrastructure for people with disabilities was really not ready for prime time when I got there in 1975. This does not mean that people with disabilities generally were not getting the services they needed. Those who had been in Berkeley for a long time were doing quite well. There was a higher concentration of people with disabilities in that small city than any other city in the world. Those who had been around knew how the system worked and how it did not work, and they had the first choice of the best personal assistants and other resources.

Those of us who were new got mostly the dregs, and the dregs at Berkeley were really dregs, the so-called "street people," who were largely vagabonds whose brains were burned out from massive quantities of illegal drugs. They were not always as dependable as one would like.

My Personal Assistants at Berkeley

The way in which many people with disabilities living at Berkeley received their needed personal assistance services—

in order to get dressed, go to the bathroom, transfer to and from their wheelchairs, get fed, and all the other things we need—was to hire people by the hour to provide such services. Therefore, like many other people with disabilities there at the time, I had to hire a weekday morning assistant, a weekday evening assistant, a weekend morning assistant, a weekend evening assistant, and assistants to help me with meals. In an average week, I would have six or seven assistants. Therefore, at the age of eighteen, I had a larger payroll than many of the small businesses in the city.

Some of my assistants were very unusual people, which is not surprising, because I was drawing largely from a population of very unusual people. A fair number of my employees were members of Eastern religions that required that they wear nontraditional clothing and conform to certain rules of behavior that some might regard as bizarre. Some of these people lived in religious communes, and many people would say that they were members of cults. I am not so judgmental about these things, in part because I have great difficulty distinguishing between cults on one hand and legitimate religions on the other. I am just happy when religious people do not try to impose their beliefs on me, and these assistants never tried to convert me. They were, without exception, very moral people, and overall they were very good and dependable employees.

I had another set of assistants who were not religious fanatics. These were primarily street people with more surviving brain cells than most of the street people. Some of them became good friends during my freshman year. One fellow named Doug was my morning weekend assistant for much of the year. This guy was continuously high on marijuana; I literally never saw him when he was not high. I certainly do not advocate the use of illegal drugs, which I believe can be very harmful, but in this particular case, I think I would have been concerned if he ever came to work without being high on pot. Being high appeared to be his natural state, and I am not sure how well he would have functioned otherwise.

I dealt with many different challenging situations concerning my personal assistants that year, including having to find emergency assistants and replacement assistants when my regular people did not show up or quit without bothering to tell me. This did not happen often, but when it did, it would be very disconcerting and disruptive. However, the most memorable incident concerning one of my personal assistants that year pertained to one of my most dependable assistants, who would have never considered leaving me in the lurch.

Mike was one of the quietest guys you would ever meet. He was my weekday morning assistant for much of the year. Every day, Monday through Friday, he would come into my dormitory room first thing in the morning at precisely 8 a.m. He would then proceed to put on one of several Bob Dylan albums and commence work. Within a couple of hours, he would have me dressed and up in my wheelchair, feed me breakfast, and take off to do his own stuff until the following workday, when he would repeat the process starting with the obligatory Dylan album.

Consequently, I would see Mike only in the mornings. But one evening, after my evening assistant had already put me in bed, Mike came running into my dormitory room, talking nonstop nonsense. I had never heard him say more than a few words in an entire morning. However, the words were really flowing out then. He then proceeded to open my big window as wide as possible and to throw his prized $500 guitar out the window. As this was happening, my dorm mates had assembled at my door, wondering what the hell was going on. With me, they witnessed Mike then proceed to go outside (fortunately, he took the long route rather than jumping out the window itself), and he finished the job on his guitar, smashing it against a tree, hopefully not in the presence of any music lovers or environmentalists.

My dorm mates and I then began debating the likelihood that Mike would show up the following day. If I were a gambling person, which I am not, I would have bet on his being there on time, and I would not have had any trouble finding people to bet against me, giving me bad odds. I would have won. The following morning, he opened the door, put on the Dylan album, and started work. Curious, I asked him, "Mike, what happened last night?" He responded, "Bad trip, man." That is all I ever learned about the incident; apparently, he had a bad experience with LSD, otherwise known as acid. Mike continued to work for me until the end of the school year without further incident.

The Disabled Students' Program

All this brings me to a somewhat sore subject. Other than the excellent academic reputation of UC Berkeley, one of the things that convinced me to go to school there, 3,000 miles away from home, was all the hype about the school's Disabled Students Program. I cannot remember whether I was part of this program during its first year or whether there was a class or two of students with disabilities before me. As I mentioned earlier, a few students with disabilities were previously housed in the university hospital, but they ultimately rebelled, telling the university that they did not want to be treated like patients or to be isolated from the rest of the students. Consequently, a new residential program was established in a dormitory. I was told that this program, which received substantial government funding, would assist me in learning how to live independently.

Unfortunately, it turned out that there were different interpretations of what it meant to assist me in learning how to live independently. My interpretation was that the program would provide support in helping me locate personal assistants, and in a difficult situation they would actually provide some emergency assistance. I thought this was a reasonable interpretation, in that the state was financing the salaries of several individuals, who previously served as personal assistants, to be available in three shifts around the clock. I figured that, as long as they were doing nothing but talking and sitting on their butts, they could help us out in the event that our assistants did not show up or if we had the occasional bladder or bowel accidents that people with disabilities sometimes have when our assistants are not available.

And, in fact, some of these workers were willing to help out under such circumstances. However, others were not. One of them in particular took the hard-line position that, if the program were not there, we would have had to deal with these problems, and therefore the best way to prepare us for our lives was not to bail us out of these circumstances. From my perspective, the problem with this "tough love" approach was that the program was there, and the state was paying for it, and these people were sitting on their butts while we were sitting in urine or worse. It seemed to me that it was not too much to ask for them to help under such circumstances. Unfortunately, he was not persuaded by this logic, nor was I persuaded by his, and due to a weak administrator, this issue was never resolved that year.

Actually, it did get resolved, in a sense; in the middle of the year, I simply stopped dealing with the program. I figured that they were not doing anything for me anyway, so why should I continue to participate in this fraud? This really bothered them, in that they were concerned that my discontinuation of their "services" could adversely affect their funding in future years. Suddenly, they could not do enough to help me. I would let them do so in some emergency situations, but otherwise I stopped interacting with the program. The only one who would still not assist me was the fellow who had taken the hard-line position against me. In a sense, I respected this adherence to principle, although I also thought that he was mostly just lazy. I was amazed, five years later, to find that he was in the same first-year class as me at Harvard Law School. This was just another one of those coincidences that seem to occur over and over in my life. We actually became friends that year, and in a way, he may have even been right to some extent. Forcing me to do it myself may have helped me in the long run; in the short run, he just made a difficult situation more difficult than it needed to be.

With freedom and rights must come responsibility and accountability.

The Berkeley Culture

There were some things I really liked about Berkeley and some things I really did not like. I liked the freedom associated with the counterculture atmosphere in Berkeley, being surrounded by artists, intellectuals, and other creative people. I truly enjoyed living in a community that accepted me, and in which I could not go down the street without seeing several people in their wheelchairs. I also liked the constant sensory simulation of this small but vibrant city.

I did not like the rampant lack of responsibility by many people in the Berkeley community. With freedom and rights must come responsibility and accountability. Although I was able to find some responsible individuals to provide my assistance, there were many people you could not rely upon. Associated with this, I believe, was an escapist mentality reflected in the constant use of drugs. I really did not understand what these people were trying to escape, in that this seemed like a fairly ideal place in which to live.

I was able to immerse myself in the Berkeley culture when, during the Christmas holidays, the university threw us out of the dormitories until the beginning of the next semester. Because I was thousands of miles from home and could not afford to fly home for the holidays, I needed to find a place to live for a few weeks. Fortunately, a very nice young lady with a disability, who lived in the community, invited me to stay in her guest room. This turned out to be an eye-opening experience.

During my stay, the entire apartment smelled of marijuana, while Joni Mitchell albums played continuously. When I was trying to get some sleep, a parade of different male and female lovers of this woman, as well as the male and female lovers of the male and female lovers, marched in and out of her bedroom. I am certainly not being judgmental, and I was probably at least a little envious, as none of them had jumped in my bed; with my luck, it would have been one or more of the males.

Although I cannot confirm this scientifically, I believe that this particular household was fairly representative of households around Berkeley at the time. Although I truly appreciated her hospitality, I was very happy to return to my dorm room after the holidays.

And There Were Studies, Too

With all the distractions of Berkeley, it was sometimes difficult to remember that the primary reason I was there was to study. On my way to class every day, I would pass by an amazing array of sights and sensations, including street performers, musicians, artists, protesters, and simply interesting-looking people. I always felt as if I were in the middle of a circus and that I was part of the show.

Remarkably, I did very well academically that year, receiving mostly As. Yet I was not very satisfied academically. Although UC Berkeley is a wonderful school for graduate students, who can benefit from personal interactions with all those Nobel Prize winners, this situation was not nearly as good for undergraduates. Freshmen such as myself were subjected to introductory courses in enormous lecture halls. I remember my Anthropology 1 class, for which I was located at the very back of one of these lecture halls. On the last day of class, the professor, who was one of the world's leading experts on African witchcraft, made a dramatic exit by walking up the steps of the stairwell and receiving an ovation. This was the first time I was close enough to actually see him, and he nodded at me briefly. At that moment, I decided that I wanted a more personal education.

As a result, at the beginning of the next semester, I applied for admission to Strawberry Creek College, an alternative school that was part of UC Berkeley. This college was designed specifically for malcontent undergraduates such as myself. It had small classes of about ten students with two professors in each class. One of the courses I took was on the subject of utopian societies. Extensive readings on this topic were required, as well as a very extensive research project. I developed a paper of over a hundred pages, which received a grade of A.

I should say a few words about how I got my work done in those days, because most students with or without disabilities nowadays seem to take for granted their computers and word processing programs. When I was at Berkeley, I was issued by New York State's Vocational Rehabilitation Services a Selectric typewriter and a mouth stick. The typewriter was a simple electric typing machine that required that each key be hit with a fair amount of pressure. A mouth stick is a simple, long piece of aluminum tubing with plastic on each side. I would put the mouth stick in my mouth and proceed to hit keys, one at a time, for hours and hours. When I finished the first draft of my paper, I would set it up on my reading stand and start the same process from scratch for the second draft. I always did three drafts of every paper, including the long paper for my Utopia course.

Moving On

Even though I enjoyed Strawberry Creek College, and it was a dramatic improvement from the large lecture halls, I still felt that UC Berkeley was not conducive to an ideal undergraduate education. I learned an enormous amount that year, but much more out of the classroom than in. After my first year at Berkeley, I believed that I could survive anything and that I could live independently.

Sensing that I was not fully satisfied at UC Berkeley, my parents came to visit me toward the end of the year and offered to check out all the other UC campuses for me. After examining many of the universities throughout the state, they gave me their report. My father seemed very impressed with all the blond women on bicycles at UC Santa Barbara.

Although I agreed that this was an important criterion, I decided that I needed to get away from distractions, not go to new ones.

I needed to find an excellent university in the UC system that did not have any distractions. My parents found the perfect school, the University of California, Riverside.

Commentary: Going It Alone in California
/Mitchell Batavia, Brother/

Drew flew the coop, a critical move in his life. And leaving home may have also been the most difficult one for our parents to handle. From their perspective, it was hard enough to let your child leave for a college 3,000 miles away but almost unfathomable to do so for a child who cannot control about 90 percent of his body. But this is exactly what they did. Had Drew remained local, he would have likely remained coddled and doomed to a lifetime culture of dependency. And who knows, perhaps he would have attended a local business school and eventually landed a job as a store manager in a stultifying mall. Interestingly, his break from family was consistent with the philosophy of the independent living movement—living with disability, independently, in the community, and outside institutions. It also allowed Drew to discover failures in the existing institutional support system for people with disabilities, which likely prompted remedies. Drew's disappointments at Berkeley with emergency assistance may have motivated him to organize a student disability organization to push for disability accommodations when he later attended Stanford University.

In a book that Drew later wrote on independent living, he argued that "one of the reasons behind the Independent Living Movement was the desire of people with disabilities to become independent of family members and friends." While it is doubtful he adopted this philosophy during his recovery at Rusk, his move to Berkeley certainly served as a catalyst. Living on his own forced Drew to rely totally on himself and consequently forced him to learn the basic survival skills for quadriplegia. It was at Berkeley that he became an adult.

In fact, our cousin Neil, who lived in Northern California at the time, would visit Drew and encourage him to be more assertive. Neil elaborates:

It was at Berkeley that he first experienced living on his own as an independent being. During this time, I saw him grow tremendously as a person taking charge of his own care and well-being. In doing so, he learned to take charge, often firing incompetent help and delegating responsibility to those who cared for his personal needs. I feel these formative experiences shaped his personality in positive ways and gave him insight into the obstacles that had to be overcome in removing barriers for people with disabilities. Once, when visiting him in Berkeley, I noticed that he had various cactuses on display. He told me that they were his favorites as they were self-sufficient and required little care.

Drew's Mannerisms

Although Drew could not move most of his body, he did have a characteristic Drew-ness that likely contributed to his charisma and became a part of his personality following his injury. I can remember his characteristic alternating shoulder shrugging to celebrate, the comedic opening of his mouth while quickly turning his head left and right to playfully express surprise, and the forward dropping of his head to express weariness.

My mother, Renée, in a fiction-writing class exercise, captured some of the mannerisms of Drew quite well:

Wearing faded jeans, a blue University of California sweatshirt, and brown corduroy cap, Drew sits comfortably in his wheelchair, his hands resting carelessly in his lap. His big, brown cow eyes are focused on his book.

The dormitory is bustling with students. Some greet him by name as they pass his partially open door. He responds with a nod, a dimpled smile, or "How're ya doing?" rubbing his goateed chin, on his chest. Periodically, he turns his head to the right; his mouth grabs a metal stick from the reading stand in front of him. He turns a page; his mouth replaces the stick in its holder.

He raises a shoulder and rubs it against his cheek

"Ready for lunch?" Joe calls, as he enters the room.

"Is the bag full?" Drew asks.

Joe puts the reading stand to the side of the room, picks up the plastic container, and empties the urine.

"Just in time," he says, adjusting the cuff of the dungaree.

Ann and Carol invite them to join them as they pass. Drew's chin works the controls diligently up and down, side to side, directing his wheels through the doorway, around the corner, and down the ramp. The motor hums as he keeps pace with his friends. Ann adjusts his cap— says it looks sexier that way.

A girl calls, "Hi, aren't you in my econ class?"

"Micro or macro?" he asks.

"Micro. See you there fifth period," she calls as she scoots by.

"Funny," he says with a twinkle in his eyes, "I don't remember seeing her in class. Wonder how she remembers me."

And Drew's twinkle was part of his charm; it was genuine, uplifting, and contagious. It helped him make friends and win arguments—and both were useful when he moved to Riverside.

Chapter 8. Then South, to Riverside (of All Places)

When I called the admissions office at the University of California, Riverside, I received an interesting response after telling the official that I would like to transfer from UC Berkeley. She said, "You want to do what?" I had to repeat the request two more times before it finally registered with her. Apparently, nobody had ever made this particular request before. Everyone wanted to go to the prestigious, interesting, and world-renowned UC Berkeley. Nobody had ever heard of UC Riverside, which was the smallest and the newest of the UC campuses. The thought of transferring from Berkeley to Riverside was practically unheard-of.

Yet this would prove to be one of the best decisions I ever made in my life. Sometimes you find the most interesting and best things in life when you get off the proverbial beaten path, and particularly when you ignore what society says is the best or most prestigious thing to do. UC Riverside proved to be the best place I could ever have received my undergraduate education. This was later confirmed through national surveys, which found that it was consistently one of the best undergraduate schools in the country. I am not sure whether it still is now, as it has grown dramatically, from approximately

5,000 students to more than 20,000 students, but back then you could get a very good education there.

Other than the university campus, Riverside is probably best known for two things: its famous Mission Inn and its infamous air pollution. The Mission Inn is a beautiful, old reproduction of a Spanish mission and was the place where Richard Nixon was married. Because I was never much of a Nixon fan, this did not impress me much, although the beauty of this old hotel certainly did. Riverside is located in a valley in the middle of the San Bernardino Mountains, where all of LA's pollution is trapped. Although this made for some wonderful sunsets, which are more colorful due to all the crap in the air, it probably reduced my life expectancy by a year or so. Even if this is so, it was worth it. My college days at UC Riverside were among the best years of my life, and friendships from that time have remained important to me throughout my life.

No Diversions Here

The great thing about UC Riverside, for someone who wants to get a good education, is that it was in the middle of a great cultural desert, and there was basically very little to do around there but study. I believe that you get your education at a university as much, or more, from your fellow students as from your professors, and I was surrounded by students who were there for all the right reasons (at least this was true of most of them). Studying was basically the only reason to be at Riverside, which did not have a beach or anything else to create a party atmosphere.

This university was very stimulating. I drove my parents a little bit crazy by breaking the world record for changing majors at a college or university. Every week or so, I would come up with a new idea as to what I wanted to do when I grew up. At one point, I was a psychobiology major, but my lack of high school chemistry put me at a distinct disadvantage. Finally, I decided upon a major of sociology, for reasons that I still do not understand, and I completed about half the coursework before discovering that sociology is the social science dedicated to documenting the obvious. At that time, I took on economics, which seemed to offer more insight, as a second major.

The Economics Department at UC Riverside, at the time, was very interesting. About half of it consisted of the traditional neoclassical economists, who taught conventional economic theory, and the other half consisted of radical economists, who conveyed the teachings of Marx, Veblen, and other unconventional economists. One professor in particular, E. K. Hunt, who had a long beard and looked particularly radical, had a significant influence on me. Throughout my four years at Riverside, he and the conservative economists, such as economic historian Roger Ransom, engaged in a competition for our young minds; I am not sure whether either side won the war, but each won important battles and influenced my thinking to this day.

At one point, I believe that my father was concerned that he had sent me 3,000 miles away to become some kind of radical revolutionary; I have since become much more conservative in my views concerning economics, though my ultimate objectives and concerns about the unfairness and inefficiency of our society remain largely the same. To those who would criticize such an intellectual transition, I would paraphrase what Judge Robert Bork said about his own ideological metamorphosis: Anyone who is not a liberal when he is young has no heart, and anyone who is when he gets older has no brain.

Throughout our undergraduate education, we had plenty of interaction with our professors. There were also many speakers who came to campus, and I attended all of these talks. I got a great undergraduate education.

My Personal Assistants

In talking about my experience at Berkeley, I discussed how I employed six or seven personal assistants a week over there. Supervising all these people turned out to be almost a full-time job. I decided to change my model for receiving assistance when I got to Riverside. I had one false start when I hired a person from outside the campus, an Eastern religious fanatic, who refused to feed me anything with any meat in it. He did not last very long. I figured out, at that time, that I was surrounded by poor students who needed money as much as I needed assistance. Also, students were more dependable than outsiders and were unlikely to tell me what I could eat.

I hired a lot of students over the next four years at Riverside, as well as a couple of outside people. I modified my situation by simply hiring one assistant for the weekdays and one assistant for the weekends. This system worked out well for everyone. Many of my assistants were premedical students, and I believe I contributed significantly to their medical educations. UC Riverside, in conjunction with UCLA's medical school, had an accelerated premed program, known as the bio-med program, in which a small number of students selected every year would automatically be admitted to UCLA's medical school and have one year cut from their overall education. A few of these students would become my assistants. I chose these individuals very carefully, and I knew that they would be excellent doctors. I did not always feel that way about some of their colleagues in the bio-med program, who I did not believe should be allowed to practice on humans.

My favorite recollection concerning one of my personal assistants at Riverside pertains to an assistant who was not a premed student. This fellow, whom I will call Colin, was my weekend assistant, was bisexual and somewhat unusual-looking, and was often hassled by some of the stupid jocks (athletes) on campus. As I mentioned earlier, I hate bullies and would always come to his defense, telling his tormentors to back off.

One Saturday, Colin was scheduled to transfer me back to bed at 11 p.m. We both had big plans for that evening. He was going to attend the hundredth consecutive showing of the *Rocky Horror Picture Show,* a musical movie with homosexual and bisexual themes in which the audience participates by dressing up and playing certain characters. Colin was in full costume that evening. My plans were of a different nature. I had a first date with a very attractive young lady whom I was hoping to impress. I took her to dinner and a movie, and we returned to my dormitory room at 11 p.m. She opened my door, only to see Colin lying in my waterbed in his wig and fishnet stockings. This is not exactly what I had in mind when I said that I wanted to impress her. I imagine that this particular mental impression remains with her to this day. After a certain amount of explanation, I think she understood, but I am not certain whether we ever had a second date.

God Save Me from Salvation

Almost all of my memories of UC Riverside are wonderful, with one notable exception. Riverside County was at the time, and I imagine still is, one of the most socially conservative counties in the country. As such, it is part of the large Bible Belt of this country, and consequently there were always many born-again Christians on campus. These people must have had some type of radar device or something, detecting that I was in the area. They would swarm upon me like locusts with the single-minded objective of "saving me." To this day, I really do not know what they were saving me from, but I know that it must have been pretty damned bad, because they were dedicating their entire lives to converting me to Christianity, an absolutely infeasible goal.

The easy thing for me to do would have been to say that I was born again and to put a serene look on my face. However, I do not do things the easy way. Therefore, I would inevitably tell them that I was either a devout pagan or a devil worshipper or something like that. (I am actually none of these, because I do not adhere to any organized religion.) Of course, such statements only strengthened their resolve to save me. So why did I do this? I guess I was just so offended that they would target me, presumably due to my disability. Some actually believed that my disability was a result of something I did wrong in this life or a previous life. I was just minding my own business, and they would descend upon me, which in my mind was simply immoral.

OK, There Were Some Diversions

Contrary to the impression that I may have created concerning the studious academic environment at UC Riverside, my friends and I were not always stoic intellectuals. This was college, and we were going to have the full college experience. I had something resembling charisma back then, and for some reason women seemed very attracted to me. At one point during my first year there, a beautiful young lady of Asian-American descent moved into my dormitory room with me. This was pretty much unheard-of and caused quite a stir at Aberdeen-Inverness Hall. I particularly enjoyed the reaction of the jocks, who could not comprehend how this guy, who was as pitiful as anything they had ever seen, was having infinitely more sex than they were (which was basically none). I think they eventually concluded that she must have been my nurse. She was not my nurse.

There were a fair number of women in my life during my Riverside years (though not as many as the 10,000 claimed by Wilt Chamberlain in his memoirs). The song "Torn Between Two Lovers" was on the radio a lot at that time, and at one point, I was in a situation in which another very attractive woman was having a hard time choosing between me and a senior who had a beard and seemed like he was a generation older than me. Again, I had the impression that he could not believe that I was the competition. Again, I really enjoyed this. It is one thing to be able to attract a beautiful woman. It is quite another thing to do so while sitting in a chin-controlled motorized wheelchair with no use of your limbs. This, to me, represented the ultimate victory over my disability. If I could compete with these guys in this particular arena, I had to be very good. I was.

I have many wonderful memories of my social life at Riverside, but my single favorite memory relates to my friend Jeanine. One weekend, the campus put on a gong show. For those who are not familiar with what a gong show is, it is basically a strange type of talent show in which the participants do not necessarily have talent (although some may). Participants perform their particular God-given talent, and the audience either applauds or boos them off the stage; at some point, the judges may hit a large Chinese gong, terminating an act before its planned conclusion. On that particular evening, there was little evidence of real talent, and most of the participants were being gonged justifiably. However, toward the end, there was an act that caught my attention.

All of a sudden, two strikingly attractive young ladies, one brunette and one blonde, got on the stage and started doing a traditional striptease act, accompanied by traditional striptease music. For the first time that evening, my eyes were focused on the stage. They proceeded to take everything off except for skimpy halter tops and panties. I had no idea what was going to come off next. Finally, at the very end of the act, both girls had their backs facing the audience and turned around, taking off their halters. Both had chests matted with an impressive amount of thick brunette and blond hair, respectively, which they had glued on. The audience went wild, applauding enthusiastically. It was brilliantly executed and one of the most creative things I had ever seen.

That is how I met and fell in love with Jeanine, the beautiful brunette girl. Directly after the act, I went up to her, introduced myself, and asked her if she would like to get together some time. That was the beginning of a beautiful love-hate relationship, which persists to this day. At the time, she was going out with one of the bio-med students, a tall, blond-haired, blue-eyed fellow with classic good looks who could have been on the cover of *GQ* magazine. I never considered myself particularly handsome—though some women, such as my wife, insist that I am in a nonclassical kind of way—and I had no idea how I was going to compete with this guy. He reminded me of pictures you would see of the kind of guys the Nazi eugenics program tried to produce, and I started referring to him as "the Nazi-looking guy," mostly to get a rise out of Jeanine (who, like me, is Jewish). She would torture me in kind.

The Nazi-looking guy ultimately won in the short run. Jeanine and I dated every once in a while and became good friends, but he remained her boyfriend for a good part of the time we were in Riverside. Years later, she told me that he once told her in referring to me, "Jeanine, never [go to bed with] a cripple!" (He actually used a more graphic term that started with the letter *f.*) I am glad that she told me this, because it is useful for me to know and understand what people are thinking and saying behind my back. It is amazing to me what they let become doctors these days! Ultimately, I won, however. Jeanine would eventually get married and raise two beautiful girls, one of whom is named after me— Emily Drew. Of all the honors I have received in my life, this was the greatest. Later this year, I will attend Emma's bat mitzvah.

Other Diversions

We had a lot of fun at Riverside. My close friends, Ann and Royce, would occasionally go with me to the campus bar, the Bull & Mouth. We also often went to a place called the Barn on campus, where great folk, jazz, and blues musicians, such as the legendary Elizabeth Cotton, played every weekend at a price that even poor students could afford. Every weekend, the campus theater played great movies, including foreign films, by directors such as Lina Wertmuller, that I loved. However, during finals week, the campus theater would play great X-rated films that had real plots, such as the story of Sodom and Gomorrah. Playing these movies apparently was intended to reduce the tension of finals. It worked!

Looking back at these finals-week movies, which were very graphic, it is truly remarkable that this happened in conservative Riverside County. These films were always very well attended; the theater would be filled to capacity with male and female students who would laugh hysterically at the ridiculous plots. No alcohol was allowed in the campus theater. One time, my friends and I put a long trench coat on a female friend of ours who was a little person, and we proceeded to sit her on top of a keg of beer, which was placed on my manual (nonmotorized) wheelchair. With the trench coat covering the keg, she looked like a giant with a tiny face and a physical disability, but nobody at the door was about to question her. We smuggled the keg into the theater. What is college without a few innocent pranks?

Finally, on some rare occasions, we would leave the campus for some diversion, such as when Ann and I and a few other friends drove down to Ensenada, Mexico, on the Baja Peninsula, and camped out on the beach. That was the first time I had been camping since my injury, and it is not so easy roughing it in a wheelchair. Although I do not believe camping will ever be one of my favorite recreational activities, we had a lot of fun down there. I still miss my old friends and the simplicity of life at Riverside.

On to Law School

I graduated from UC Riverside with honors. During my senior year, I had to decide on the next step to take. One possibility was to enter "the real world." This did not seem very appealing. Getting some entry-level job based on my bachelor's degree was not going to pay for my extensive expenses. Clearly, I needed to become some type of highly overpaid professional. In the absence of any clue as to which profession to pursue, I followed the time-honored approach taken by thousands of clueless graduates. I took the LSAT and applied to several of the top law schools in the country.

My first choice was Stanford Law School, which seemed to me the ideal place to attend law school. I was placed on the waiting list at Stanford. In the meantime, I was accepted at Harvard Law School. I was excited that I was accepted into one of the top schools in the country, but I was also a little concerned that I would freeze to death in Massachusetts. I waited until the very last day permissible to accept the offer from Harvard, hoping that Stanford would come through in the meantime. When the deadline came, I contacted Harvard immediately, telling them that I was honored to accept.

A Triumphant Return

Fifteen years after I received my undergraduate degree, and soon after I had worked in the White House, the Justice Department, and the Senate, UC Riverside Chancellor Raymond Orbach took me to Washington, DC's famous Cosmos Club, of which he was a member. This was one of the most prestigious social clubs in the nation's capital, its walls lined with pictures of Nobel Prize winners who are also members, which gave the place the feeling of gravitas. During lunch, the chancellor invited me to deliver the commencement address for the UC Riverside graduation ceremony in 1995 (see Appendix C). This was one of the greatest honors of my life, and it was particularly meaningful to me to be speaking at my alma mater, the school I truly loved, that gave me the best undergraduate education one could receive. The next thing I knew, I was back in Riverside, staying with Cheryl, who was by then my wife, at the Mission Inn.

During the commencement ceremony, I was awarded the university's highest honor, the Chancellor's Award. This medallion, which was placed around my neck during the ceremony and now resides in my home office, was previously awarded to only seven other individuals, including President Gerald Ford. I delivered my commencement speech twice, to audiences of about 10,000 people in each of two ceremonies, one in the morning and one in the evening. Speaking to this many people is really an experience. Although I kept waiting for the butterflies to arrive in my stomach, they never did show up. I received two standing ovations. A member of the university administration later told me that this was the first time in his recollection that a commencement speaker had ever received a standing ovation.

Chapter 9. Then East, to Harvard Law

The very name of Harvard, or "Hahhhvahhd" as some of the Massachusetts natives pronounce it, elicits an immediate response in the minds of most people who hear it: excellence, tradition, prestige, power. Harvard Law School is the oldest continuously operating law school in this country, established in 1817. I arrived there a little later, in August 1980. When I was growing up in New York City, the giant skyscrapers always made me feel big; I suppose I felt that I was part of the species that was able to achieve this monumental task. For some reason, the much smaller buildings at Harvard, and the place itself, had the exact opposite effect on me—they made me feel small. It is not that I did not enjoy being there, which I did in many respects, but it had this strange diminutive effect that I had never felt before. I should probably not admit this, but I have a strong commitment to honesty, a trait that is not always rewarded in our society and has precluded any prospect for my pursuing a political career.

I believe the law school experience generally, particularly at places like Harvard, is designed to have this humbling effect. I was one of many people who had passed through these halls, and some much greater than myself had distinguished themselves in this place. I am not sure how many of my fellow students were having similar thoughts, but

I imagine that some did. The movie and TV series *The Paper Chase* and the popular book *One L* (the term for us first-year law students) portrayed the humbling and sometimes intimidating nature of the first-year experience at Harvard. It turned out that, by the time I entered the law school, things were not nearly as oppressive as they were in the old days. Still, just being in the same place as all these ghosts had to make you feel somewhat insignificant and make you wonder whether you were up to the challenge.

I suppose my reaction may be excused, to some extent. I was one of the first students with a major disability admitted to Harvard Law School, and mine was the most substantial mobility disability to that date (to the best of my knowledge). I have never considered myself handicapped, in the general sense of the term that means disadvantaged; however, not being able to use one's arms or hands in this particular context, before the information age, was something of a handicap. I understand that several years earlier, the guy whose life inspired the play and movie *Butterflies Are Free* graduated from this law school even though he was blind. Obviously blindness presents all sorts of other challenges for law students, who are required to read extensively.

I was going to get through this, but I was not at all certain how. I did not always enjoy the process, but I got through it just like everyone else; actually, it was not just like everyone else, but I got through it as well.

Welcome to Harvard Law

When I first arrived at Harvard, I received my dormitory room assignment, Story Hall, one of several law school dormitories named after distinguished Harvard jurists. Story Hall, honoring the renowned jurist Joseph Story, was about fifty yards from the law school cafeteria, which I would soon learn was attached to all the other law school buildings by an elaborate tunnel system. Therefore, during the winter, all that I would have to do was to transport myself those fifty yards in order to get to my classes. Since I arrived in the late summer, this did not seem like an impossible task.

I felt differently about this short commute one day in December, during a particularly bad first snowstorm of the year. My wheelchair got stuck in a snowdrift on the path to the cafeteria; within minutes, I was converted into a disabled snowman. However, this particular unpleasant experience, from which I was rapidly rescued and eventually defrosted after several hours in the company of an electric heater, was not a big deal and was more amusing than anything else (at least after I defrosted).

When I arrived in Cambridge, Massachusetts, initially, it was deceptively sunny and warm, and we were being treated (although our tuition actually paid for it) to a very nice picnic on the law school grounds. I remember the famous Professor Alan Dershowitz, who had already established a national reputation as one of the top criminal lawyers, introducing himself to me and some of my new friends. I appreciated this friendly gesture from a member of the faculty, particularly one who indicated that he was originally from Brooklyn, like me. I was a little concerned that he was the only professor I remember being at this function, but it was primarily for the students to get to know one another, and I was rapidly developing friendships.

Pertaining to friendships at the law school, I was informed by one of the second-year students that the previous year the dean of the law school had told the following story: Two Harvard Law students were out camping together and were confronted by a large bear. One of the students started running as fast as he could. The other student started laughing and said, "Don't be foolish, you cannot outrun a bear." Without stopping, the running student replied, "I don't have to outrun the bear; I just need to outrun you." The dean then proceeded to tell the entire 1L class that they should look to their left and their right, because one of those two students would not be there the following year. So much for friendships at the law school, I was thinking. I was just happy that the dean chose not to repeat that charming story in my first year.

Section 4: Leaving the Best for Last

It turns out that I did develop several long-term friendships that year. Around the time of the picnic, I was informed that I would be in Section 4. At that time, Harvard Law School admitted a 1L class of about 600 students, who were divided into four sections. Each section had about 150 students who shared the same schedule and took the same courses together from the same professors. Consequently, your section is where you were most likely to get to know people best and where you were most likely to develop lifelong friendships. In the second semester of the first year, and in the following two years, students can take a broad array of electives, in which they have classes with other students and professors, but the first year is such an intense, bonding experience that the people in your first-year section are very important to your law school experience.

Once again, this was another one of those rare circumstances in which good luck actually kicked in for me. Section 4 was a great section. I am sure that people in other sections also thought that theirs was the best, and I hope that their experience and friendships were just as good. However, even without considering my fellow students, there are reasons that one would want to be in Section 4, and many students in other sections expressed their dissatisfaction that they were not with us. Some even petitioned the law school administration to transfer to Section 4. Much to their further dismay, they were denied this request.

Probably the primary reason people wanted to be in our section was that we had Professor Arthur Miller for civil procedure. During the first year, all students took the standard required curriculum of contracts, tort law, criminal law, property law, and civil procedure. The latter, which addressed the various rules and processes for conducting a civil case, was arguably the most important course for litigators, and Arthur Miller was the most renowned civil procedure professor in the country. His flamboyant style, in which he would interrogate students using the Socratic method while walking a couple of miles back and forth throughout the lecture hall, was legendary. You may recognize the name of Professor Miller as a result of his popular legal-issues TV shows that were broadcast during the 1990s. Before one class period, he was walking around the classroom, stopped and stared at me for what seemed to be an eternity, and proclaimed, "I like to wander." I just figured that if you are as good as he is, you can afford to be a little idiosyncratic.

The other Section 4 professors also were wonderful, although some were more wonderful than others. Among my favorites were Professor James Vorenberg, who taught us criminal law and would become dean of the law school the following year, and Professor Todd Rakoff, who taught us contracts and demonstrated a real sense of caring for his students. Although the classes were typically very serious, there was also a lot of joking. Some of our fellow students were talented actors who would write and perform great skits in which they would parody the professors and fellow students. While some of these depictions hit fairly close to home, everyone accepted them in good humor.

My Classmates in Section 4

What really made Section 4 special, however, were my fellow students. I cannot even begin to describe the remarkable cast of characters in our class, and in mentioning a few, I will no doubt offend the many I do not. However, a few deserve special mention due to the long-term friendships we established or for other reasons. If you have discerned that I have a distinct preference for members of the female gender, you would be correct. Therefore, I will begin with them.

One of my favorite classmates from day one was a young lady named Tina. I gave up any romantic notions concerning her very early, when it became obvious that every guy in our class wanted to marry her. She had the triple advantages of being very smart, very beautiful, and very nice. Tina ultimately married a very good guy named Marc, who graduated first in our class. Cheryl, the woman who would become my wife about ten years later, and I would attend their wedding, as they would attend ours. They probably still do not know that their wedding had a key role in getting us together.

Another wonderful woman in our section I will mention, at the risk of alienating all others, was my friend Silda. She is a Southern belle from North Carolina, and similarly smart and beautiful. With her Southern charm, Silda single-handedly raised the classiness of our section. She eventually married another Harvard Law graduate, Eliot Spitzer, who would later have a distinguished political career, which has included serving as the attorney general of New York State and prosecuting the massive corruption of Wall Street.[1]

Anne was another remarkable woman from the South, whose father had once been the governor of Virginia. We became good friends in contracts class, where we sat next to each other; it is amazing to me how the serendipity of a seating chart can impact one's friendships for life. Anne would later become a well-respected judge in her home state. Her husband, Timothy (Tim) Kaine, another Harvard Law graduate from another section that same year, would later be elected mayor of Richmond.[2]

Diane, another very smart woman, could easily have had a career as a model. She is strikingly attractive, with beautiful blond hair, which made debating with her very challenging. It is important to be able to focus when you are arguing complex legal issues, and it was not always easy to focus when debating with Diane or any of these young ladies. I suppose that everyone has some Achilles' heel, and this is mine. I am fairly sure that I was not the only one with this particular weakness. Diane ultimately married Robert Bork Jr., the son of the famous jurist and an accomplished writer in his own right.

All four of these close female friends would become excellent lawyers. The fact that three out of four of their husbands were also Harvard Law students is evidence that there was more than just studying going on when we were in law school. Dating fellow law students seemed a little too incestuous for me, and the thought of marrying an attorney was not particularly appealing, in any event. Most of my relationships at that time were outside the law school, to the extent that I had time for much of a social life in those years.

Despite my tendency to discriminate against male people, a few of them also deserve special mention. One fellow, also named Marc, was renowned for his radical critiques of our social and economic institutions. He was one of the most cynical people I have ever met, and I liked him very much. The other individual, whose name is John, is one of the most conservative thinkers I have ever met. Although we did not become close friends at the time, I always appreciated him.

At Harvard Law School, which is an extremely liberal place, those who expressed conservative views often were hissed by the other students. Although this was usually done in good fun, it always offended me to some extent. I admired John because he was never deterred by the ridicule and would often espouse some conservative gem that would inevitably elicit a reaction. Interestingly, he and I would eventually serve in the Justice Department of the first Bush administration, though he was always infinitely more conservative than I was at my most conservative. He is now a conservative law professor, and we disagree on most issues, though I will always appreciate his intellectual honesty.

Of course, no Harvard Law class would be complete without a Roosevelt or a Kennedy, and we even had one of these. Although I did not get to know him well, Mark Roosevelt, who, I believe, was President Franklin Delano Roosevelt's great-great-grandson or something like that, was in Section 4. Although I probably would have preferred that he be a descendant of Theodore Roosevelt, my favorite president, one cannot be too choosy about these things, and I should be satisfied that there was a Roosevelt in our class at all. I was actually one of the people responsible several years later for ensuring that Mark's ancestor was appropriately portrayed in his wheelchair in one of the statues of his memorial in Washington, DC, correcting an intentional oversight by the memorial's planners, and I am very proud and inspired that one of our greatest presidents had a major disability.

Finally, I should also mention that the other three sections no doubt had some equally remarkable people. I already mentioned that my old antagonist from the Berkeley Disabled Students' Program, was in our first-year class that year. Another fellow who was a teaching assistant in one of my freshman courses at Berkeley was in another section of our first-year class. And there were many others whom I never got to know but I am sure have gone on to brilliant careers in or related to the law. With apologies to the other members of my first-year class, all of whom contributed to the remarkable experience, space limits my ability to mention all of them.

1L: A Challenging Year

When I look back at my first year at Harvard, I must admit that it was challenging; there was an enormous amount of information that needed to be absorbed and integrated in a relatively short period of time. I believe that it was challenging for virtually all of us, although I am not sure that all of us would admit it. All of us, without exception, were accustomed to being among the top students, if not the top student, in every academic setting in which we had ever been. It is somewhat daunting to be competing with an entire class of students of our same caliber, some of whom had truly remarkable intellectual capacities.

I use the word "competing" carefully, because in one sense we were really competing and in another sense we were not. By virtue of having been admitted to one of the top five law schools in the country—each of which, of course, contended that it was the top school—we were all going to get decent jobs practicing law. Therefore, unlike the situation of law students in virtually every other law school in the country, who were not guaranteed good jobs, we were not really competing with one another. Whenever my undergraduate students tell me that they want to go to law school, I always tell them that they had better get into one of the top schools in the country or they had better be close to the top of their law school class, because otherwise they may not find employment in the law. My classmates at Harvard and I did not have that concern, and therefore the dean's charming story about running from the bear was mostly just hype.

In another sense, however, we really were competing. Each of us was accustomed to being among the top, and most of us were committed to staying there, even in this rarefied atmosphere. I was not exempt from these delusions of grandeur. Being at the top of Harvard Law School meant making the law review. The *Harvard Law Review* is arguably the most prestigious academic law journal in the country. It is run by student editors, who are considered the elite of the law school. Editors of the *Harvard Law Review* inevitably got many of the very best jobs, including clerkships with respected judges and sometimes even clerkships with Supreme Court justices. Making law review could make your career.

There were two ways to become an editor of the *Harvard Law Review*. First, you could be selected as an editor if you had among the highest grades in your first-year class. Second, you could be selected as an editor if you entered and were among the top competitors in a legal writing competition. Anyone could enter this competition, which was held in the spring semester of the first year. I convinced myself that the last thing I wanted to do was to spend the next two years of my life checking on the references cited by arrogant law school professors. The grades I received at the end of the first semester were pretty much average, which meant that the only way I could make law review would be through the writing competition.

Therefore, I was somewhat upset with myself when I found my wheelchair, accompanied by me, in line with all of my fellow students when the time came to pick up the case that was to be analyzed for the writing competition. I suppose that my delusion of grandeur raised its ugly head and forced me to line up with the others for the honor of becoming subject to the last vestige of slavery in our country—the *Harvard Law Review*.

Fortunately, I came to my senses a few hours later after reading the case and learning that it involved an analysis of an exception to the automobile exception of the Fourth Amendment right to be free from unreasonable searches and seizures. This was arguably my least favorite issue in my least favorite subject, criminal law. I was not about to spend a week of my time researching it, with a remote possibility of beating out all these other smart people, some of whom actually liked this issue. I promptly threw the papers away, and with them any hope that I would be on the *Harvard Law Review*. I felt relieved immediately.

The only greater feeling of relief I experienced that year was learning in June 1981 that I had passed all of my first-year courses. This meant that, two years later, I would graduate from Harvard Law School. I received average grades, just like almost everyone else I knew. By that time, this did not bother me much. I had survived the experience with my dignity and several new friendships, and that was good enough for me.

2L: The Harvard Law Employment Agency

Once you made it through the first year of law school at Harvard, you were basically a lawyer. This does not mean that you knew an enormous amount about the law. Even after the third year at one of the top schools, your knowledge of law is still largely rudimentary; it takes years of practice immersed in the law to actually become knowledgeable of it, and senior attorneys and law professors are always learning. This is in part because there is so much to know and in part because the law is always evolving as our society evolves. However, by the end of the first year, assuming that you have survived, you are going to be an attorney.

Consequently, starting at the beginning of the second year, Harvard Law School and all the other top law schools become large legal employment agencies. Dozens of employers would come to the campus, trying to get the best students to accept jobs in their law firms, corporations, government agencies, and, in a small number of cases, public interest organizations. Although students still had to take and pass their courses, there was no doubt that if you did not voluntarily drop out, you would graduate. Overall, people were much less concerned about their classes than their job prospects. Virtually everyone ended up getting a job, though some students were more happy than others about their offers.

The way this employment thing worked was that employers—particularly the large law firms considered most desirable by students, in part because they paid the most money—liked to hire 2Ls for summer internships in which they could determine whether they wanted to hire the individual on a full-time basis. Representatives from the law firms and other employers would come from all over the country to interview the Harvard Law students.

Students could sign up for as many interviews as they wanted, and the employers could not choose which students they wanted to interview. This created an interesting situation for me. The employers did not know about my disability prior to my interviews, and some of them would probably have been happier if I had not signed up for them. It would often be apparent to me, within a few minutes into the interview, that the employer had no intention of ever hiring me; usually, the glazed look in their eyes was the giveaway.

Of course, this was about eight years before the Americans with Disabilities Act of 1990 (ADA) was enacted, and therefore they could have discriminated against me overtly without breaking any law; in other words, they could have just said to me, "You look like you would be a lot of trouble, and we would rather not have to accommodate your needs." However, saying this would have been very poor form and would have created ill will with the law school.

Therefore, the prospective employers were all very cordial and friendly to me. When the time came to give offers, however, most of my fellow students received many while I received only a couple. The good news is that you only really need one, and I received an offer of summer employment with one of the top Wall Street firms, Fried, Frank, Harris, Shriver & Jacobson.

I mention the firm of Fried Frank by name because they deserve a lot of credit for being able to look beyond my disability at my abilities. I had never been subject to discrimination before, and it did not feel great. My fellow students with identical academic records were receiving ten times as many offers as I was. Fortunately, I could not have done any better than Fried Frank. The Shriver in the name of the firm was Sargent Shriver, the famous Democratic politician. The firm was initially established by Jewish lawyers who could not get jobs with the big WASP law firms, which discriminated against them. When they hired me, they had no idea that I was Jewish, as my name is not a traditional Jewish name. I had a great summer with them; all of us summer interns were wined and dined and not required to do a lot of work. At the end of the summer, they extended an offer of employment to me.

And There Were Classes, Too

Other than seeking employment during my second year at law school, I have few recollections of the year, with the exception of two courses. I remember I took constitutional law from Professor Larry Tribe, the premier liberal scholar on that subject in this country. Professor Tribe would lecture without referring to notes for two consecutive hours in the giant lecture hall in Langdell Hall. This was an extremely popular class as a result of Tribe's national reputation, and an overflow of students would be sitting on the stairs.

As he lectured brilliantly, that lecture hall became warmer and warmer, as the body heat of all the students accumulated. Unfortunately, the only wheelchair-accessible seat in the hall was approximately five feet in front of Professor Tribe; every day, approximately forty-five minutes into his lecture, I would fall asleep directly under his nose. No matter how much coffee I drank prior to class, I could not prevent my eyes from becoming heavy and heavier with every word, until they ultimately closed. Fifteen years later, when I was involved as an attorney in a Supreme Court case with Professor Tribe on my side as the lead attorney, I was hoping that he would not remember this.

The one other second-year course I remember was administrative law, because it was taught by Professor Byse, who, according to the gossip within the law school, was the model for Professor Kingsfield, the character in *The Paper Chase*. Whether or not this is accurate, Professor Byse was approaching the end of his career by the time I took his course, and he had apparently mellowed quite a bit by then.

Even at his fairly advanced age at the time, he was still sharp as a tack intellectually. That was true of all of our professors. Although I did not necessarily admire all of them as people, one had to respect and appreciate their mental capacities and their accomplishments.

Off to the Harvard of the West

I cannot really say that I enjoyed Harvard Law School; it would probably be more accurate to say that I appreciated it. However, I would not have wanted to do the first two years of law school anywhere else. Although I thought that I wanted to be admitted to Stanford for my first year, I believe that the intensity of experience at Harvard was more interesting and important to my development. It may not have been as pleasant as Stanford, but it had a major impact on me. Never again would I feel small or insignificant wherever I went, no matter how imposing the institution.

Ironically, I got to study at Stanford anyway. By the middle of my second year at Harvard, I desperately needed a break from law school education. I really felt that legal education was not terribly intellectually stimulating, and I had a desire to learn new things. I wrote a letter to Professor Victor Fuchs, who is based at Stanford and was probably the top health economist in the country. This set off a process by which I was eventually admitted to Stanford, sometimes referred to as the Harvard of the West.

Commentary: Paying for School
/Mitchell Batavia, Brother/

Higher education comes with a hefty price tag, and Drew must have racked up a bucket of student loan debt, having gone to both Harvard and Stanford.

Our mother never recalled taking out student loans for Drew, so it was a bit of a mystery how he was able to afford the top schools in the nation. She did serve as his private social services center and was pivotal in locating resources for him. For example, Drew received much assistance from New York State's Vocational Rehabilitation Services. And certainly SSI benefits for students with disabilities helped. In addition, there may have been scholarships, although this is pure speculation.

But evidence that he took out loans and paid them all back can be found in a thank-you letter to President Reagan. Drew wanted to demonstrate that, given the opportunity, people within the disability community can be valued, contributing, taxpaying members of society. All he really wanted, I believe, was to have what you or I have in a democratic society: opportunity.

Drew loathed pity, eschewed welfare, and clearly never wanted to be a burden, much less institutionalized. His antipathy for charity is illustrated in the following story that took place in New York City during a well-paid Wall Street law internship while he was attending Harvard Law. Drew, our parents, and his personal attendant spent an afternoon in Washington Square Park back in the summer of '82. With its famous arch and circular fountain, the nine-acre park—once a farm, gravesite, and parade ground—sits at the foot of Fifth Avenue and is the cultural crossroads of Greenwich Village, complete with musicians, chess players, street entertainers, revolutionaries, and hot dog vendors. Our mom and attendant purchased a soda, placed the plastic drinking cup on Drew's lap, and then went back to buy some hot dogs. While this was happening, an elderly man who was passing by tapped Drew on the shoulder, whispered, "God bless you," and dropped a dollar bill in the plastic cup. Drew, mortified, called out, "Mister, you come back here right now and take this back." The man turned briefly, waved to him, blew him a kiss, and kept walking. Drew kept calling, "Come back here" until the man was out of sight and lost in the crowd.

Chapter 10. Back West to the Farm: Stanford Med

I like to tell people that I graduated from Stanford Medical School, which is accurate. However, if I ever gave doctor's orders for people to take off their clothes, stick out their tongues, and say "ahhh," I would be arrested for practicing medicine without a license, or at least I should be arrested. My degree from Stanford is not an MD degree, but rather an MS degree in health services research. The decision to pursue this degree was another one of the best decisions of my life. This is not because it gave me substantially greater earning power, which it did not; my intellectual pursuits have actually cost me a lot of money over time. What it did was give me a unique perspective that most lawyers do not have, which has been valuable for me throughout my career.

Just being at Stanford was wonderful. I believe that Stanford is the greatest university in the world today, although thinking this obviously is in my interest. It is also one of the most beautiful. The campus is replete with Spanish-style buildings with orange tile roofs; large green areas outside are sprinkled with Rodin sculptures, such as *The Thinker,* throughout the campus. Unlike Harvard, which was a wonderful but somewhat stoic experience, Stanford was a wonderful and joyous one. Students, who would refer to

Stanford affectionately as "the Farm," because it was originally on a farm when Leland Stanford decided to locate his university there, would walk around the campus with smiles on their faces.

I was among the most happy of all; I had experienced Harvard, and now I was experiencing Stanford. One could hardly be more fortunate in one's lifetime.

The Lifestyle of a Graduate Student

In my view, there is no better life than that of a graduate student, particularly at Stanford University. The climate is perfect, the setting is beautiful, and your job is to learn as much as you can about the field of study that you have personally chosen. Unlike being an undergraduate, you presumably know something, though not a lot, and you have access to some of the finest minds (of some of the finest people) in the country. What more could you ask for out of life?

If, in fact, there is no better life than that of a graduate student, there was no graduate student at Stanford who had a better life than me. I had a great apartment, which was really a little house, in the graduate student housing at Stanford. There were four of these little houses adjoining one another, with a courtyard in the middle. My neighbors were other graduate students from a variety of different fields, some of whom were married and had children, unlike myself at the time. Some were international students. It was a great group of people.

Stanford was very good to me. It provided my first of many automatic door openers, which gave me the freedom to come and go as I pleased. I was always coming and going to and from campus for classes and other activities. To me, this was heaven.

However, this pleasant situation was being experienced by all of the graduate students living in the graduate student complex. So why did I have the best life of all? That year, I hired as my personal assistant a Chinese fellow named Li, who, remarkably enough, was trained in France as a chef. Every week that year, he prepared a large pot of the best French onion soup I ever tasted, which I ate for breakfast for seven days. One might ask whether I ever got tired of eating French onion soup for breakfast. The answer is no. I could eat French onion soup every morning for the rest of my life. Every evening, he would prepare a different gourmet meal, and he never prepared the same meal twice. The aromas would inevitably permeate the surrounding student houses, and the level of envy was more than perceptible and growing. Occasionally, I would invite my neighbors for dinner, in part so that I could share my good lifestyle with them and in part so that they would continue to speak to me.

During one spring break, Li and his ninety-year-old mother, sister, and I took a road trip circling around the southwest United States, stopping off at several interesting places, including Las Vegas, the Hearst Castle, and Death Valley. His mother and sister did not speak more than a few words of English, and yet we were able to somehow communicate with one another. We must have been quite a sight to those watching us. However, we had a great time. Life was very good!

My Early Career as an Activist
My good lifestyle should not suggest that all was well for people with disabilities at Stanford in 1982. In some ways, the university was exemplary, as evidenced by the way in which it provided me with my accessible apartment and automatic door opener. Yet, in other ways, it was not as good.

Probably most disconcerting to me and several of my fellow students with disabilities is that the undergraduates, in particular, seemed very sheltered and tended to ignore our presence on campus. Also, there was no official university policy for accommodating the needs of people with disabilities, and therefore university efforts to accommodate our needs tended to be very ad hoc and not always consistent.

Probably the best piece of advice I could give a young student is to seek a good mentor.

A small group of graduate students with disabilities, including myself, established a small student organization, which we called Stanford Disabled Students (SDS). The fact that we had the same acronym as a prominent radical group may have been somewhat disconcerting to the university administration. I was elected president of SDS, and we proceeded to request a meeting with Dr. Donald Kennedy, the popular president of Stanford University. Dr. Kennedy graciously met with us, listened to our concerns, and established a university committee to address our concerns. I served on a committee, and we established the first comprehensive policy on disability for any private university in the United States.

The Two Tall Economists of Stanford

At the time I was going to school, the two top health economists in the country were at Stanford: Victor Fuchs and Alain Enthoven. Both of these men stood well over six feet three inches tall and were tall in every sense of the word. From a wheelchair, the physical height of these men was itself somewhat daunting, in that I had to tilt my head up higher than I was accustomed simply to converse with them. This greater physical distance seemed in some ways symbolic of the enormous distance between what they had achieved in their lives and what I had achieved in mine. In my defense, they were both in their early fifties at the time, and I was twenty-five years of age. Still, the distance in knowledge and accomplishments seemed almost insurmountable.

Probably the best piece of advice I could give a young student is to seek a good mentor. A mentor can provide very good advice to keep you on the right path and to avoid unnecessary problems and diversions. I had the best mentor in the country.

As I indicated, I had written to Victor Fuchs when I was a second-year student at Harvard. I had known about Professor Fuchs as a result of having read his landmark book, *Who Shall Live?*, which was required reading in an undergraduate course on health care at Riverside. This book changed the way I thought about public policy. I knew when I read it that I needed to learn more from this man. My second year of law school was the ideal time to contact him. I told him that I was bored intellectually and that I wanted to study under his guidance.

Alain Enthoven was based at the Stanford Business School. I took two courses in which he was a professor and learned an enormous amount from him. When I was there, he was just developing the theory of managed competition in health care, which became extremely influential and served as the basis for the Clinton administration's health care reform plan (before the proposal went out of control and developed a life of its own). As with Fuchs, I spent a fair amount of time before and after classes trying to absorb everything I could from this man.

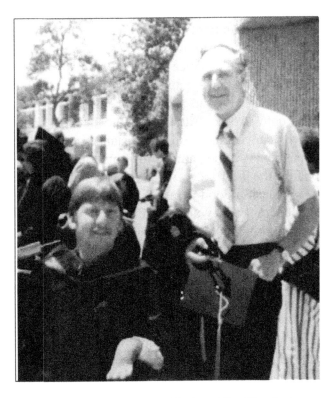

Drew with Professor Victor Fuchs at the Stanford commencement.

One day, Professor Enthoven made the most generous comment that anyone ever told me in my life. I cannot remember the specifics of our conversation, but at one point he said that he wished that he was smarter than he was. He went on to say that he believed virtually all professors felt that way about themselves. For some reason, this was a revelation to me. Here, one of the smartest men I had ever known, who was one of the McNamara "Whiz Kids" at the Defense Department during the Vietnam War, who was frequently asked to serve as a consultant to government and top corporations, and who was my professor at the top university in the world, had just said he wished he was smarter. Remarkable!

Although I continued to believe that Alain was definitely smart enough, this comment somehow made me feel closer to him.

The Program

The health services research program was a highly interdisciplinary program in which students could take appropriate courses throughout the university. Moreover, the students themselves were from a variety of different fields. This was my educational ideal: the opportunity to interact with people from a broad array of different professions, disciplines, perspectives, and orientations, and with a variety of skills, methodologies, and value systems. This was the exact opposite of what I had just experienced at Harvard, where I was dealing with lawyers and law students virtually all the time.

I truly enjoyed and appreciated this program. It was precisely what the doctor ordered to cure my intellectual boredom. In looking back at it, this experience raises images in my mind of how the most fortunate students were educated in ancient Greece, where they discussed issues with teachers like Socrates, Aristotle, and Plato. Although law schools always like to talk about how they use the Socratic method, which involves professors asking probing questions about cases that are assigned, my experience in the health services research program simulated the real Socratic method. I remember thinking that I needed to absorb every word Victor Fuchs ever told me. He conveyed to me the greatest gift a teacher can convey: the standard of excellence that I would take with me for the rest of my career and my life. This experience was about as close as one can get to that classical experience nowadays.

Other than the informal exchanges between the students and professors, my favorite aspect of the program was the ability to participate in the symposium series. This was a set of presentations by distinguished scholars and practitioners throughout the country who would assemble in a lecture hall in one of the oldest buildings of the medical school. There would always be one individual presenting the results of his or her study, and everyone else in the audience prepared to raise questions for and comments concerning the presentation. Students were encouraged to participate actively, and I would occasionally raise a question. What would always happen is that the more people talked, the more confused the issue became, and an almost palpable fog would develop in the lecture hall. Then, toward the very end, Victor Fuchs would stand up and talk for a few minutes, and the fog would dissipate, and everything made sense all of a sudden. I always thought to myself, I want to be able to do that.

Toward the end of my master's year, I presented my thesis on the academic medical center under the new Medicare Prospective Payment System and was pleased that my thesis defense took place in the same lecture hall as the symposium series. My audience was not large but made up in quality what it lacked in quantity, and the presentation was well received.

Graduation

There was one additional small piece of business that I had to attend to before leaving Stanford, not that I was in a hurry to leave. I still had to finish my third year of law school. All of my friends who had been in Section 4 with me at Harvard had graduated in 1983, the year I did my master's.

Therefore, there was really no sense in going back to Harvard for my third year. Moreover, I had this vague recollection that it was very cold back there, and it was very pleasant at Stanford. I had already visited Stanford Law School and asked if I could do my third year there. The fact that I was willing to pay the Stanford tuition in addition to 10 percent of the Harvard tuition made both institutions happy and amenable to my doing the last year at Stanford Law School (as a Harvard law student attending Stanford).

That year was valuable to me for a couple of reasons. First, I was able to compare two of the top law schools in the country. For some reason, while the professors at Harvard were always fighting with each other, those at Stanford with very similar ideological differences worked together peacefully and in a constructive manner. It taught me that organizational culture and environment are extremely important. Second, I was able to do my major third-year paper, which is a requirement for graduation at Harvard, under the guidance of Professor William Baxter. Baxter was the top public official in the Antitrust Division of the Justice Department during the Reagan administration. He was responsible for breaking up the AT&T monopoly, possibly the most important antitrust case ever. My third-year paper on antitrust issues in the health care field was ultimately published in a major law journal.

In June 1984, I celebrated my graduation from both the health services research program at the medical school and from law school. My wonderful parents and grandparents came all the way out to Stanford to be with me. My grandfather was appalled that I would not wear a tie. However, I refused to yield on this based on principle (wearing ties violates my personal religious convictions), and in any event, you could not see it under the cap and gown. At the Stanford law graduation, I was the last student to be called to the podium. They announced "Andrew Batavia, JD from Harvard Law School, MS from Stanford Medical School." Nobody in the audience except for my family knew why I was even on that particular stage that day, but I got a standing ovation anyway.

Another Triumphant Return

I returned to Stanford on two occasions since I graduated. On the first, I attended the retirement party of my mentor, Victor Fuchs. I was one of the few of his students to be honored with an invitation, and this occasion was very special. A full day was dedicated to a discussion of Vic's many contributions to our knowledge. By this time, I was no longer a student, but rather a very junior colleague of his as well as a friend, and I remained as impressed with him as the first time I met him. The concept of this occasion being a retirement party is a little misleading, in that he has remained as productive as he was prior to "retirement." He did retire from the classroom, which was a loss to his students, but this has given him the additional time and flexibility to pursue his research and discuss it in his travels. I would not have missed his send-off for the world.

On the second occasion, I had the honor of representing the White House at Stanford's centennial celebration. This was also very special to me. I had the opportunity to present the first Bush administration's perspective on health care reform as part of an expert panel on health care issues. Also on the panel was Professor Alain Enthoven, who was my professor of health care policy and one of the most brilliant and influential economists in the health care field.

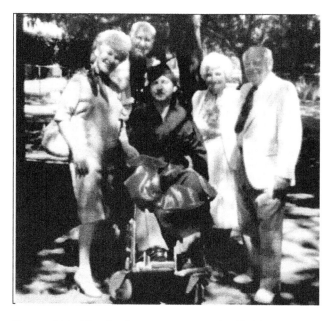

Drew at his Stanford commencement with his
parents, Renée and Gabriel, and his grandparents,
Anne and Joe Hyman.

Throughout the three-day celebration, Stanford treated me as
a VIP, providing wheelchair-accessible transportation and
accommodations for wherever I wanted to go. I attended a
celebratory dinner attended by many dignitaries and
celebrities, including Tom Brokaw (the NBC news anchor). It
does not get any better than this!

The First Medical Crisis
/Mitchell Batavia, Brother/

To graduate from two of the top schools in the nation was an amazing intellectual milestone for Drew. But 1984 also heralded his first medical crisis since his car crash. That summer he suffered from a major infection while he traveled in his van from Stanford to the East Coast by way of Canada with an attendant. I say "major," because he had had minor, low-grade infections on and off since his accident. I was in Toronto at the time, taking a course, when he dropped in to see if I could take him to the nearest emergency room. Not being that familiar with the Toronto health care system, we were first turned away from an ER because it was for pediatric care only. Eventually, we found an adult ER, where he was placed on a gurney, examined, and prescribed antibiotics for his first serious urinary tract infection. Unfortunately, it would not be his last.

Chapter 11. A Government Paycheck: Achieving Brain Death

When I extended my education at Stanford, the firm of Fried, Frank, Harris, Shriver & Jacobson extended its offer of employment for an additional year. This offer was very tempting. I cannot remember the exact dollar amount, but I do remember that it was a lot of money at the time, more than I could earn anywhere else in the economy. For a person with very expensive needs, including the need to employ a full-time personal assistant 365 days a year, it is difficult to turn down such an offer. It is particularly difficult to turn it down when the people extending the offer have been extremely nice and decent to you. Yet I did turn it down.

This was the first of several times during my career that I turned down big bucks to pursue the job of my choice; all together, I estimate that I have forgone a couple of million dollars so far in my life that I really could have used, and still could use, for that matter. Often, when people say this, it is out of some self-righteous sense of superiority concerning "selling out" or becoming part of the establishment or some similar nonsense. I do not adhere to these ideas. Generally, I have nothing against the big law firms or corporations per se, though I certainly do have objections as to how some of them have conducted themselves in the recent scandals. Yet, the majority of these organizations are run in an honest and honorable manner, and in some ways I wish that I could have joined these organizations, because it would have made a difficult life somewhat easier.

I turned down the generous offer of Fried Frank because I felt that I really had no choice. It would have been unfair for me to accept their offer, because I could have never given all of myself to the firm. Such law firms are basically hired guns for any client who has a desire and resources to retain them. Again, there is nothing wrong with this. From a technical perspective, it presents real challenges to attorneys to provide the best possible representation for their clients. Such clients deserve their best efforts; however, they did not necessarily deserve my best efforts. I needed a mission in which I believed deeply. Without such a mission, I could not give all of myself. Fried Frank and its clients deserved better than what I had to offer. I appreciated that they did not make me feel any guiltier than I felt already. These were good people who were good to me.

Finding a Mission with the Federal Government

Not being able to accept the law firm offer still left a fundamental issue: How would I make a living with a paycheck large enough to pay my bills? This would have been much less of an issue if I were independently wealthy, which I am not. Working for one of the few public interest organizations that conducted interviews at the law schools would not have paid the bills. Moreover, I was not altogether convinced that many of these public interest organizations actually represented the broader public interest, to the extent that there is a discernible public interest.

For example, although I support most of the overall premises and goals of the American Civil Liberties Union

(ACLU), I do not always support their specific positions on issues or their selection of clients such as neo-Nazis and Ku Klux Klanners. They always argue that they do so because the important thing is the issue—protecting our First Amendment rights—and sometimes you have to protect the rights of the most despicable to preserve them for the rest of us. Although I was persuaded by this argument philosophically, as well as the argument that everyone deserves legal representation, again, I did not feel that they deserved my representation. Moreover, those who buy these arguments generally have a fair amount of faith that our legal and political systems will ensure that the right party prevails. I do not have the faith.

I needed a mission that provided a paycheck. In other words, I needed something that I thought I could believe in that would still pay the bills. I found this in the federal government. The Office of the General Counsel of the US. Department of Health and Human Services conducted interviews at Stanford during my third year of law school there. I was impressed with them, and they seemed impressed with me. To them, my disability was actually a plus, in that they were always trying to find qualified people with disabilities to serve in the federal government. Finding someone like myself, who had gone to the very top schools, must have been a godsend to them.

I received an offer soon after my interview. The amount of the offer was about 50 percent less than the offer from the law firm, and the differential would grow dramatically over time. This notion of taking a virtual vow of poverty was somewhat painful to me. However, at least I would be working in the health care field, and I would be representing the interests of the public. Or so I thought.

The Great Hall

The Hubert Humphrey Building on Independence Avenue in Southwest Washington, DC, houses much of the top administration of the Department of Health and Human Services. In our nation's capital, many people seem to be fixated on stupid things such as access to power. Therefore, the closer you were located to the office of the secretary, the chief federal official appointed to this department by the president, the more symbolic access you had. My office was not even based in the Humphrey Building. It was across the street in a much older building that was built during the Great Depression and had wonderful murals from that period that were created by artists participating in the Work Projects Administration. I actually enjoyed being in that building, and I had no objection to being about as far away from access to the secretary of Health and Human Services as I could be.

I cannot say that I was exempt from thoughts about the trappings of power in Washington. Just about every time I was in the Great Hall of the Humphrey Building, I would pay my respects to the portraits of the secretaries that were displayed around the walls. The secretary, the chief executive officer of the department, is appointed by the president and confirmed by at least a majority of the Senate. For some reason, I had developed a great deference for these individuals. At the moment, I can't remember precisely why I held them in such esteem back then.

Part of this one-person fan club was justified by the quality of such individuals as Elliot Richardson, who had distinguished himself in many years of government service and in many ways, but who is probably best known for when he served as President Nixon's attorney general and refused to fire the special prosecutor, Archibald Cox, during the Watergate era. Other secretaries had also distinguished themselves through years of public service. One of my favorites was Joe Califano, who served as one of President Lyndon Johnson's chief aides and helped to establish Medicare and Medicaid. He later served as secretary of the Department of Health, Education, and Welfare under President Carter (this was about the only thing I liked about the Carter administration). However, in retrospect, I believe that much of my admiration was based largely on the naivete of youth and the awe associated with the big boss.

In any event, I started developing career fantasies of serving as secretary at some stage of my career. If I had shared these thoughts with any of my colleagues at the time and told them that I would like to be secretary, I am sure they would have asked me how many words I could type in a minute. If, in fact, I had such lofty aspirations, I was certainly starting at a strange place. I was starting at the department as a mere staff attorney. Although this was a professional position, and attorneys did have some stature in the department's hierarchy, it was about as low a professional position as one could have as an attorney. The distance between myself and the secretary, in terms of power, influence, or compensation, could not have been greater, and my prospects for these things could not have been much less.

I remember during Christmas of 1984, my first year at the department, that I waited on the receiving line to exchange holiday greetings with Secretary Margaret Heckler, who was appointed by President Reagan. After about an hour, I made it to the front of the line and had a picture taken with the secretary. When the picture was developed, she very graciously personalized it with her signature and the following message: "Thank you for your excellent legal work in helping to implement the Medicare Prospective Payment System."

Someone from the secretary's office actually called my supervisor and asked what I had worked on. I was impressed that Secretary Heckler would take the time from her busy schedule and that of her staff to do this for me. I wondered whether it was done because I have a disability or whether everyone who requested a personalized photo received one. Whatever the reason for this gesture, I thought it was a very nice thing to do, and it motivated me to work harder. It taught me that small acts of thoughtfulness at the highest level can have a major impact on morale at the lowest level.

The Benefits of Disillusionment

The somewhat naive notion I had at the time that the government represents the broad interests of the public deserves some further examination. It no doubt emanates from the philosophies I absorbed while growing up among the liberal, Jewish middle-class, which basically believed that government is a force for good. I still think this can be true, depending largely upon which public officials are in power and which political forces are being exerted at any point in time. However, irrespective of the current administration, there are a variety of institutional issues that ensure that the broader public interest will not be adequately represented in political or legal processes.

Based upon substantially more experience, I now believe that the broader public interest is likely to be respected by high-level government officials primarily in crisis situations in which the press and the public eye are focused on what these officials are doing. Otherwise, special interests and the particular ideological interests of the officials are likely to prevail. Those interests that can afford to contribute, financially and otherwise, to the political process, and can afford to hire expensive lawyers and lobbyists, are much more likely to get what they want when the public is not looking closely.

Precisely how political factors would play out depended, in part, upon the specific administration in power and who was in bed with that administration. The Reagan administration was dominated by officials who did not trust federal employees and wanted to downsize the federal government to the fullest extent feasible. Of course, they would say that doing so was in the broader public interest. A careful analysis of their policies did not always reveal such laudable intentions. At my lowly level, however, I did not have much perspective on these abstract philosophical issues. I just basically helped to implement what they had decided to do. These decisions were made at a much higher pay grade.

The Work of a Government Staff Attorney

There were three main components of the work of attorneys at my level at the Department of Health and Human Services. I worked in one of the divisions of the department's Office of the General Counsel, whose clients were several agencies, the largest and most important of which was the Health Care Financing Administration (HCFA). This agency was recently renamed the Centers for Medicare and Medicaid Services (CMMS). Other clients included the Administration on Aging and the Office of Developmental Disability Services.

Reviewing Proposed Policies

With respect to the first component of the attorney's work, when the client agency wants to develop a new policy, the attorneys are typically asked to review the proposed policy to determine whether it is legal. This was one of the things I did most, and I was very good at this. The reason I liked this work was that I consider myself more a policy person than a legal analyst. In fact, when I went to law school, it was with the primary objective of becoming a policymaker. This was also why I took an additional year to get my master's in health services research from Stanford Medical School.

What much of the public does not understand is that a good legal education can provide a strong general background for a lot of different careers, including a career as a policymaker. My parents certainly did not understand what I was doing. They just figured that if you go to law school, you practice law. I was actually doing that during my first job at the department, but I was also getting some of the policy experience I wanted. When I was reviewing an agency's proposed policy, I felt as if I were participating in the policymaking process. Although I was not hired to provide policy advice, I occasionally did so as a participant in the process.

I was asked to review a proposed policy to cover heart transplants under Medicare. From a policy perspective, this did not seem to me to be a great idea, in part because the heart transplant technology was still relatively new at the time and in part because many more beneficiaries would have been assisted by increasing coverage of other, more cost-effective technologies. However, my job was to provide legal advice, not policy advice, and I wrote the legal memo that authorized the coverage of heart transplants under Medicare. Specifically, I concluded that coverage could be limited to those centers that provide the most transplants, based on empirical evidence that patients were more likely to survive and benefit from the procedure in those centers. It was good legal work, and the department was not ever successfully challenged concerning this policy.

Reviewing Regulations

The second component of the government attorney's work involved promulgation of regulations. Often, when a government agency wanted to implement a new policy and the attorneys determined that the proposed policy was permissible, the agency would then have to develop a detailed regulation to implement the policy. This was not as simple as one would think. The primary purpose of the regulation was to give everyone who could possibly be affected by it an opportunity to comment on it ahead of time, so that the agency could be aware of all concerns and possibly modify the regulation before implementing it. This involved a very complex, multistage process in which the agency would have to develop a notice of proposed rulemaking, and in which the regulation is published in the *Federal Register* for public comments. Later, a final rule is published incorporating whatever changes the agency adopted. Usually, the rule itself was only a few pages long, but the material accompanying the rule, explaining it and why the agency did not modify it, often went on for dozens or even hundreds of pages.

Before any of these proposed regulations or final regulations could be published, they would have to be reviewed and approved by the attorneys. That was another of my specialties. For each of these regulations, I would receive a draft that was typically about 300 to 400 pages long. The draft regulations were mind-numbing in their level of boredom. The attorney with the onerous task of reviewing these regulations would have to go through them word by word, sentence by sentence, and paragraph by paragraph until every aspect of the regulation was scrutinized. I was one of the very few attorneys there who had the capacity to endure such boredom.

Now, I imagine that you are thinking, didn't I say that I had a low threshold for boredom? Yes, you are absolutely correct, and this paradox requires some explanation. I am bored whenever I am doing something that I do not regard as important or as a good use of my time. Conversely, I am not bored whenever I am doing something that I regard as important or a good use of my time, even if what I am doing is itself the most tedious task on this planet. Reviewing those regulations was arguably the most tedious task on the planet Earth that year, and yet I found it exciting, which gave me the motivation to trudge through the thousands and thousands of words in those regulations. Some of those regulations were necessary to implement Medicare's new Prospective Payment System, which was why Secretary Heckler commended me for my work.

Litigation

The third component of the government attorney's work was representing the department and its agencies in litigation. No matter how good a job we did in reviewing proposed policy and developing regulations, the department would be sued by individuals or organizations that felt they were adversely affected. I actually think a lot of these lawsuits lacked merit, and some are absolutely frivolous, brought with the hope that they could extract a settlement. Often it is in the interest of the agency being sued to settle a claim out of court rather than expend enormous resources in defending a lawsuit.

From the perspective of many of my colleagues, one of the most attractive aspects of government work was the opportunity to argue in court at an early stage of your career. At the big law firms, very few associates have a chance to argue cases in their first couple of years; many must wait until their third, fourth, or fifth years, or even later, and are relegated to litigation support until then. This is because the clients of these firms pay hundreds of dollars per hour for hundreds or thousands of hours to be represented by these firms, and they would not be very happy to know that young associates right out of law school were getting their litigation experience at their expense. The federal government, with its enormous number of cases, could not afford this luxury, and virtually any young attorney interested in litigation could take on as many cases as he or she wished, practically from day one. Some of these attorneys, who became very good litigators with an expertise in this particular area of health care law, cashed in on this experience later in their careers by switching sides and joining law firms that specialized in suing the department.

I was not one of the attorneys who was attracted to the opportunity to litigate. I always thought of litigation as a somewhat nasty affair, which at best was a necessary evil and at worst was an entirely avoidable waste of valuable resources. I somehow had developed the novel notion that, if policy issues were handled appropriately and different parties operated in a reasonable and civil manner, most litigation could have been avoided entirely. I have learned recently that, since the time that I graduated from law school, this notion of preventing and avoiding litigation has been labeled "therapeutic jurisprudence." This, like so many other things in our society, amuses me; we seem to need a name to label and thereby legitimize common sense. Still, we should probably be grateful that such common sense has been given some legitimacy in that it flies in the face of the prevailing American norm: When in doubt, litigate.

Several of my closest colleagues at the department were litigators. These were very smart and capable people who are also very good and ethical people. Yet when they were in litigation mode, they were very aggressive and sometimes pugnacious people. I think that the litigation process has that effect on a person. You almost have to take on that demeanor, because litigation, at its most basic, is a fight between the heroes of each party, not unlike the Colosseum fights among gladiators in ancient Rome.

The outcomes of such litigation often involve large sums of money, typically involving between tens of thousands and millions of dollars. If the clients of the firms were not satisfied with their representation, there were always many other firms from which to choose. Consequently, the private attorneys tended to be very aggressive, requiring the government attorneys to be at least equally aggressive in response.

Although I had no desire to become a litigator, it seemed to me that if I was going to be an attorney, I should have some experience in litigation. This is actually a wise thing to do, in that you really cannot be very knowledgeable about avoiding legal train wrecks unless you have been involved in resolving such wrecks. Litigation is a legal train wreck; it is what happens when everything has fallen apart and there is a need to put together the pieces, or at least compensate those who have been harmed. In this context, people were harmed financially rather than physically, or at least that is their contention. I asked my supervisors if I could have a few cases to give me this important experience. Initially, this was a very good thing that snowballed into a very bad thing.

My Mini-Career as a Litigator

My litigation career started out well enough. I had one case in federal district court in which I had to argue that the department was justified in limiting payment to a Medicare provider on the basis of the reasonableness of costs incurred. This case only involved a few tens of thousands of dollars, and I won. I was also involved in some litigation concerning state Medicaid eligibility requirements. Again, the department prevailed in these cases. This notion that I won these cases itself deserves a certain amount of explanation.

Litigators often make claims concerning their winning records. Some legends, such as Roy Black and Johnnie "If it doesn't fit, you must acquit" Cochran, have been created, in part, based on their winning records. There is no doubt in my mind that these are good attorneys, but I am not as certain that they are as good as they think they are. We must recognize that whether an attorney wins or loses a case depends more upon the circumstances of the case and the resources of the clients than the skills of the attorney. Of course, a great attorney can make all the difference in a very close case, but overall, win-loss records are not the best indicator of lawyer competence.

Keeping the Secretary out of Jail

One case I will never forget for the rest of my life involved the so-called "disproportionate share" requirement under Medicare. This is a requirement under the Medicare program whereby the statute requires that the program provide certain extra compensation to health care providers that serve a disproportionate share of patients who are Medicaid recipients. The department was required under the statute to develop a formula for compensating these providers. Unfortunately, the department chose to ignore or delay, for a substantial third time, the development of this formula until well after the statutory due date. Finally, after being frustrated with what they regarded as delay tactics for an extended period of time, the providers sued Secretary Heckler in her official capacity for contempt of Congress.

There are several bad things that can happen to a federal attorney, but certainly high on this list would be to have your chief official thrown in prison. This was one possible outcome if the secretary were found in contempt, and this was not a very attractive outcome. I am not even sure whether I had known that the secretary could be found in contempt of Congress. It is important to note that the secretary's predicament was in no way the fault of myself or any of my colleagues. In fact, we had warned department officials on several occasions that they needed to develop this formula that was required by statute. Still, this would not have mattered much if, at the end of this litigation, the secretary had to change residences to the big house.

My big mistake was to tell my supervisors that I wanted more litigation.

Although the typical hours of a government attorney are basically 9 a.m. to 5 p.m., any semblance of what is typical disappears in the event of a crisis. This situation was a crisis. For the next fourteen days and evenings, I was in my office working on our legal brief, which presented our arguments in writing. To make matters worse, the policy official responsible for developing the formula was scheduled to be at an important conference that weekend, and insisted upon being at that conference. I could have required him to cancel the conference by going over his head to his supervisors, but I did not want to do this to him, and I allowed him to go to the conference. If we had lost the case, that decision would have been held against me. Fortunately, we were able to assemble a strong brief, allowing the judge to resolve the case without depriving the secretary of her liberty.

Of course, we were aware at the outset that it was not likely that a federal judge would actually throw the secretary of DHHS in jail. However, the very possibility of this was enough to cause enormous stress and require me to lose two weekends in which I would have preferred to be places other than my federal office. At the end, though, we survived the ordeal with only a slap on the wrist and a requirement that we develop the formula by a specified date. This time, the department had learned its lesson, and rather than being cited for contempt of Congress after all this, developed and implemented the formula. I suppose it was an interesting experience, and one that reinforced my belief that I did not want to be a litigator. If there was any doubt at all about this decision, it was resolved in another case in which I was at fault.

My Mea Culpa: I Screwed Up

My big mistake was to tell my supervisors that I wanted more litigation. I should have left well enough alone. The department was involved in some mass litigation in which almost every provider in the country sued the department for its policy. The best example of this occurred when the department decided that it was no longer going to pay for the malpractice insurance of Medicare providers. The department probably could have achieved this objective but would have had to publish this policy in a formal regulation in the *Federal Register*. Instead, in an effort to save hundreds of millions of Medicare dollars, the department decided to attempt to do this retroactively, initially with no regulation and later with a regulation that was to be applied both retroactively and prospectively.

As a result of these decisions by high-ranking federal officials in the secretary's office, the department had virtually hundreds of cases brought against it to invalidate the new policy and require the department to pay malpractice insurance costs. Privately, several of my colleagues and I agreed that the department had acted poorly in developing this retroactive policy. However, we had no choice but to defend it. Each of the attorneys had to handle a fair share of this litigation. This was a miserable task because, unlike my other individual cases, which involved a lot of intellectual and creative work, these cases simply involved modifying certain boilerplate language to fit specific circumstances. This was extremely boring and unsatisfying. Moreover, I did not feel as if I were part of an honorable mission. Therefore, I grew to despise this work.

Still, this does not excuse what I did. After one of these cases was decided against us, I failed to apply for an appeal of the decision. This was very bad, and I learned this very soon. As soon as the department learned that it had to pay up, its officials were irate. Apparently, the department's strategy was to try to delay payment as long as possible by filing appeals and motions. My screwup really interfered with these plans. For the next week or so, I was subject to a modern version of the Spanish Inquisition. Although I indicated that it was my understanding that the Justice Department automatically filed appeals in all of these cases, I also indicated that I was willing to take full responsibility for the error, even if it meant losing my job.

You would think that this would have ended the matter. It was not as if I had done something intentionally wrong. I did not do anything that would have enriched or otherwise benefited myself. However, there were a couple of supervisory attorneys of the female persuasion who were intent upon making me feel as bad as possible about this situation, indicating that it was tantamount to malpractice. I suppose they were right, but this does not mean they had to abuse me verbally. Nothing they could have said would have made me feel any worse than I already felt.

I mention that my tormentors were female primarily because this was very surprising to me. I had always gotten along very well with members of the female gender, and I still do. However, this was my first employment situation in which women had supervisory responsibility over me, and they were much harder on me than my male supervisors. Interestingly, in the two other situations in my career in which I have had problems with other employees (neither of which have involved fault on my part), the individuals causing the difficulty were female. I have since heard from numerous female coworkers that they strongly prefer having male supervisors.

After sufficient abuse by these two supervisors, and I really believed that this amounted to verbal abuse at this point, I pointed out to these attorneys that the fault was not all mine. Young attorneys like me, right out of law school, had received no training or guidance whatsoever from the Office of the General Counsel. There were no systems whatsoever to ensure that things like this did not fall between the cracks. Although I was willing to accept responsibility, I was not willing to accept all the responsibility. They were equally to blame, though they never would have admitted it. Mostly, they just enjoyed pointing downward, which allowed them to preserve their crappy little careers.

Federal Brain Death

In my mind, I have conceptualized four categories of attorneys who worked with me at the department, and that I assume would apply generally to other government professionals at this department and other agencies of the federal government. For lack of better terms, I will refer to them as the following: the appointees, the lifers, the traitors, and the escapees. To satisfy any curiosity you may have at the outset, I became an escapee. I am glad that I got out when I did.

The Appointees

The appointees were a small number of individuals who attained their positions through political appointments either from the White House or the department; often there are conflicts between the White House and the secretary as to whose people will receive an appointment. Sometimes the secretary is saddled with one of the president's friends or supporters whom the secretary does not know and has not chosen. However, most presidents allow their agency heads to surround themselves with most of their own people. The appointees have relatively high-ranking positions that typically involve policy-making or other decision-making authority.

The notion of a federal political appointment sounds very impressive and imposing. This is because when the press addresses political appointments, it is inevitably referring to the highest-ranking appointments, such as cabinet officers. What the public does not see typically are the multitude of lower-ranking appointments. When a new president is elected, his (or theoretically her) chief personnel officer is flooded with tens of thousands of resumes and cover letters of individuals, some of whom donated fifty dollars to the presidential campaign and therefore feel entitled to a government job in the new administration. The skills and qualifications of these individuals vary dramatically, from exceptional to nonexistent.

Whether a qualified person received a position depended upon a variety of factors, including their skills, their relationships, and the amount of their contributions. It may have also depended to some extent upon which political party was in power, but I did not stick around long enough to study this systematically. I arrived at the department in September 1984, which was in the midst of the Reagan administration. Given President Reagan's avowed disdain for the federal government, and my assessment that he was not the brightest guy in the world, I had anticipated that his appointees in the department would not be a bunch of savants. This proved true to some extent, though there were also a few very intelligent and capable people in appointed positions. Which officials fell in which category, I will not say at this time.

The Lifers

The lifers were those attorneys who decided to make federal work their career. Some did this by design, deciding in law school or at some other time that they wanted to be government attorneys for as long as they would work. This was not a completely irrational decision; although government work does not pay a fortune, working conditions and benefits tend to be good. I worked under the assistant general counsel, one level under the general counsel, who is the chief legal adviser to the secretary. At this level it was rare to find many attorneys in their offices after 5 p.m. on weekdays, and attorneys were virtually never in their offices during weekends.

While some of these attorneys planned, from the outset, to stay with the government, others simply woke up one day and realized, "Oh my God, I am a lifer." It is understandable how this might happen. Working for the department was a relatively comfortable life, and the federal retirement system at the time was fairly generous, with defined benefit pensions based upon the number of years at the job. If you stayed twenty years, you would receive a fairly hefty pension and still be relatively young. This notion attracted me momentarily, until I came to my senses. I thought that being a lifer would certainly be better than looking back from your deathbed at a career that yielded a lot of money and little else to show for it. Still, being a lifer would have been as boring as hell and could not offer the real sense of mission I needed.

If I had decided to stay in the federal government, I definitely would have attempted to join the Senior Executive Service. These were the elites in the federal civil service, who are paid the best among the nonappointees and who had the greatest responsibility. Two of these fellows were among my favorites in the department. Michael,[1] a brilliant fellow, was a graduate of Harvard Law School, like myself, though he graduated about fifteen years before me. He had a big sign on his door that said, "Never ask a pig to sing. It won't work, and it annoys the pig." I never knew quite how to take this, but I assume that it was not meant as a compliment to me or my coworkers.

One of the most amusing things about being in that office was watching Michael and another senior attorney named Alan, both of whom were Orthodox Jews, walk up and down the corridors together talking loudly about arcane issues of Medicaid eligibility. It reminded me of a painting my grandfather once painted of several religious people gathered around the table, yelling at each other about arcane points in the Jewish Bible. I really liked these guys, and I learned a lot from them.

Finally, two characteristics concerning Michael that relate to his lifer status are worth discussing. First, he would always leave the office at precisely 5 p.m. I could be engaged in a conversation with him concerning work issues, and at 5 p.m. he would take off, even if we were in midsentence. I suppose I could understand this, because he made a deal with himself whereby he was willing to forgo the big bucks in exchange for a reasonable schedule. He was not going to allow anyone to modify that schedule.

Second, whenever anyone would escape to another job, we would always have a small party to wish our colleague well. Virtually everyone would contribute to the gift, with the exception of Michael. Again, I could understand this in that it must get old, spending what little money he was paid to purchase a gift for yet another person who was escaping, while he would never escape.

The Traitors

The traitors were those attorneys who developed their legal skills, particularly litigation skills, with the federal government only to join the private sector, typically with a powerful law firm. Perhaps the term "traitor" is somewhat harsh, in that there is certainly no obligation to stay with the federal government, and moving back and forth between the public and private sectors is a time-honored tradition within our system. Some would say that this is a good thing, because it results in a cross-fertilization of ideas and skills; others would say it is a bad thing that reflects the inherent corruption of our system of governance.

I suppose that I could even be accused of being a traitor to some extent, in that I had swerved in and out of government throughout my career and, at one time, was with a big law firm for a couple of years. However, my concept of a traitor is much more specific, involving specific actions in which the skills and knowledge obtained in the federal government are then used against the federal government. The very idea of defecting to a large law firm so as to litigate against the department directly after leaving is something I would not have considered.

The Escapees

I was basically an escapee. This is a residual category consisting of those who did not stay permanently and did not defect to the opposition. This was the proverbial road less traveled, which is often the more interesting road but also the more challenging one. This certainly proved true in my life.

Escape to the Private Sector

After the failure-to-appeal fiasco, I was pretty well demoralized. My demoralization was partly the result of my failing to meet my own professional standards, but much more a result of the failure of the administration to support me when I was in need of their support. This is an overstatement, in that a few of my supervisors were very empathetic and supportive throughout this difficult period, and virtually all of my lateral colleagues—the attorneys with positions similar to mine—were very supportive. However, many in the top level of administration really let me have it. At times, I thought that my career was over.

In retrospect, such thinking was foolish, in that the amount of the loss to the taxpayer was infinitesimal, considering levels of departmental spending and the fact that the federal government wastes more money in a minute's time than I had lost in that case. Yet, I can understand why I felt this way; it is easy for a young attorney to lose perspective after screwing up. I imagine that some get sufficiently depressed that they become ill or even contemplate suicide. I never fell to that depth, but I definitely was depressed. Supervisors should be very sensitive in dealing with or reprimanding their young employees. Most of mine were not. Fortunately, I had a strong support network and was able to recover from this episode fairly quickly. By this time, my future wife, Cheryl, was with me, and she helped me work through these issues in my mind.

Even when I was at peace with my failure, I continued to resent the process by which I was interrogated and reprimanded, and I wanted to get out as soon as possible. My escape hatch turned out to be both another federal agency and a private not-for-profit organization. The federal agency was the National Institute on Disability and Rehabilitation Research of the Department of Education, which sponsors the Mary E. Switzer Research Fellowships. This was a one-year fellowship to conduct research on some area of disability-related research. I somehow hooked up with Dr. Gerben DeJong, the director of the research center. With his guidance, I developed a proposal to conduct research on the financing of medical rehabilitation services. I was awarded a Distinguished Fellowship and published two books and several articles. Most important, I had escaped the federal government without too much damage.

Chapter 12. The Private Sector

Republicans like to characterize the private sector in idyllic terms, as if private organizations, and particularly corporations, have some quasi-magical properties. On the other hand, some on the Far Left, such as Ralph Nader, tend to characterize corporations in a manner suggesting that Satan himself was either on the board or had negotiated agreements with the board of every corporation in this country. I never bought into this anticorporate mentality. By the time that I left the federal government, I was ready to experience for myself the private sector of the American economy.

OK, I did not experience the full brunt of the private sector at this time. The National Rehabilitation Hospital (NRH) in Washington, DC, and the research center associated with it, are nonprofit corporations. Many economists nowadays have concluded that in the current, highly competitive economic environment, nonprofits conduct themselves and perform much like for-profit corporations. But it is certainly true that nonprofits must always be focused on the bottom line these days, lest their costs exceed their revenues, forcing them to close their doors to the public. Still, the fact that the operators of nonprofit organizations officially are not permitted to inure to the benefit of private interests creates at least the perception, and I believed to some extent the reality, that they are interested in more than just the bottom line.

The National Rehabilitation Hospital

NRH was established in 1986. It is the youngest of all the medical rehabilitation centers in our country, and it was the first and only such center established in the nation's capital.

The visionary who founded NRH is a man named Ed Eckenhoff. He is a person with paraplegia who uses a manual wheelchair and who can get around to some extent using crutches and braces, much like my friend Susan at Rusk, where I did my rehabilitation. You remember Susan, don't you? Actually, Susan was prettier than Ed, but Ed did have other redeeming features. One of those features is that he is a very hard worker. This impressed me for a variety of reasons. First, I am always impressed by someone who has a mission and pursues it with great vigor, as Ed pursued the establishment of NRH. Second, I am always particularly impressed when such individuals pursue their missions despite adversity, as Ed did even when his body started to deteriorate from the strain of using his crutches. Third, I am even more impressed when the individual has the resources not to work but does so anyway out of a desire to make a contribution. As I understand it, Ed has the advantage of being from a family with substantial wealth, and yet he resolutely refuses to stop working, years after his planned date of retirement.

Another of Ed's features that I respect greatly is his confidence in himself. His vision was to establish and build the finest medical rehabilitation center in the world. To take on this challenge in an extremely competitive environment, he made a commitment to attract the very top people in the field. Space does not allow me to discuss all the remarkable people who have worked at NRH during its formative years, but suffice it to say that they are a veritable *Who's Who* of the rehabilitation field.

Again, a couple of people deserve special mention. The NRH's current medical director, John Toerge,[1] is one of the top rehabilitation doctors in the country. He deserves special mention, in part because of his leadership role in the acute hospital, and in part because he has managed to help keep me alive over the years during a variety of acute crises to which we people with quadriplegia are occasionally subject. Dr. Lauro Halstead is another excellent physician, one who has a disability resulting from polio. He deserves additional mention because he is a member of the board of directors of my own nonprofit organization, AUTONOMY, Inc., which will be discussed later.

It is a tribute to Ed that he was able to attract the best minds in the field. This included the person who was responsible for bringing me on board, Dr. Gerben DeJong.

My Friend Gerben

I first met Gerben by telephone when I was working as an attorney in the Department of Health and Human Services. I am not sure exactly how I learned about him, but I believe someone told me that this was someone I needed to know. At the time, I was dying to make my escape from the department. The challenge was how to achieve this.

At the time I contacted him, Gerben was already considered one of the premier health services researchers dealing with disability and rehabilitation issues in the world. I say "in the world" because he had already, in his midforties, achieved an international reputation. This was expedited by the fact that he was born in the Netherlands, where much of his extended family still lives, and he is very well connected throughout Europe. However, the primary reason for his reputation is that he is simply the best researcher in the field. His work is extremely broad in scope, but he is best known for his work on independent living and documenting the independent living movement. Despite these accomplishments, I had never heard of him, mostly because I was practicing law, and we were working in different fields and socializing in different circles.

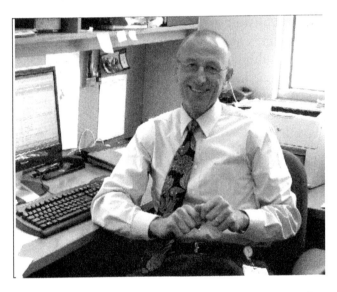

Gerben DeJong, director of research at the National Rehabilitation Hospital in Washington, DC, where Drew and he jointly wrote twenty-five published articles to bring attention to the health care needs of individuals with disabilities. Four of these articles were reprinted.

Just as I had never heard of him, Gerben had never heard of me. There is no reason that he would have, as I was just a staff attorney at the department who had not really accomplished anything of note at that time. I had graduated from Harvard Law School and received my master's from Stanford Medical School, which seemed to impress him. Gerben was always looking to recruit researchers with disabilities, recognizing that personal experience with a disability can provide invaluable insight into such issues as what needs to be studied and how to best study it. I am sure that he had never met anyone with my particular combination of background and credentials. Almost immediately, he wanted to bring me on board. Unfortunately, he could not do this without resources, and NRH did not have any hard funding available at the time.

This notion that researchers serve as agents of social legitimization, which I had never really thought about before, was very powerful to me.

Consequently, the only way I could make my escape to NRH was if I could obtain grant funding to do so. At Gerben's suggestion, I developed a proposal for a Distinguished Fellowship with the National Institute on Disability and Rehabilitation Research to study the financing of medical rehabilitation services. This was somewhat frustrating, because I could not get out of the federal government soon enough. My only good option for doing so offered no guarantees and would not allow me to leave, if at all, until several months later, when the proposal was accepted. Fortunately, it was accepted, ultimately, and I was awarded a Mary E. Switzer Research Fellowship by the US Department of Education. My career as a rehabilitation researcher began.

Gerben has influenced my life in many ways, including allowing me to change my career and thereby change the course of my life. One of the ways he affected me is by changing my attitude toward research. My master's degree was in health services research, so I knew a fair amount about research methodologies in the health care field. Still, I looked at research from a fairly cynical perspective; I still do now, for that matter, but for different reasons, which I will discuss later. My cynicism at the time focused primarily on what I perceived as the poor quality of much of the research I reviewed. Gerben convinced me that it was possible to conduct good research in this field, and that the very act of studying rehabilitation and meeting the health care needs of people with disabilities helps to legitimize these issues and needs in our society.

This notion that researchers serve as agents of social legitimization, which I had never really thought about before, was very powerful to me. This seemed like a worthy mission, possibly not forever, but at least for a period of time. Both Gerben and I recognized that, if we were going to help to legitimize this field, we would have to do rigorous work and the results of this work would have to be published in the best journals. Gerben had already published fairly extensively in the health care, rehabilitation, and policy literatures; even I, at the age of twenty-eight, had published a few articles. In the next two years at NRH, I published two books and several monographs, and Gerben and I jointly published more than twenty articles.

My Escape from Research

At this point in this book, the astute reader has probably identified at least one flaw in my character, that I do not like to stick around the same job for too long. I actually warned you about this tendency up front, when I indicated that I have a low threshold for boredom. This characteristic, which I do not regard as a flaw, often manifests itself in a need to take on new professional challenges. By this time, I felt I had already done the research thing, at least at NRH, and I was ready to do something new.

In my defense, I believe that this is, at least in part, an issue concerning the need to learn. Once you have been in the same organization doing the same thing for a period of a couple of years, you have already learned much of what that organization can teach you. Therefore, I think it is advisable, and I often advise my students to change organizations and careers every once in a while, when they feel as if they are stagnating. In addition to enhancing your lifetime learning, this strategy, if done well, can improve your earning potential, provide a more satisfying and dynamic career, and prepare you for situations in which such changes are actually forced on you externally.

Due to my nature, I took my own advice to what some may regard as an illogical degree. I do not regard it as such, though I would understand why some may. I was becoming the disabled equivalent of Houdini, escaping to my next job as soon as I had derived what I thought I could from the current one. In this particular situation, I was motivated much less by the need to get away than the desire for an exciting new opportunity: to serve at the highest level of the federal government.

Commentary: A Conflict of Interest?
/Mitchell Batavia; Brother/

One area of Drew's work troubled me. It was his dual role as both a health policy researcher and a disability activist. Was there a conflict of interest? It was a question I pondered ever since I became aware of his activism. From my perspective, it seemed incompatible for Drew to be both; the latter would eventually sway the former. And the potential for bias is omnipresent in the research community, as most of us have a pet theory or favored hypothesis. I never had a frank discussion with Drew on this issue, even after we started writing together.

However, I was relieved to discover that Drew actually published a paper on this topic titled "Representation and Role Separation in the Disability Movement: Should Researchers Be Advocates?"[2] In his paper, Drew described the cautious role of policy researchers when their job during an analysis was only to point out strengths and weaknesses, consider alternative policies, and identify assumptions, evaluation criteria, and value judgments of proposed policy. Thus, their role was to analyze, not advocate. In fact, Drew believed readers should draw their own conclusions. He also viewed it as highly suspect for someone to maintain a role as analyst and at the same time lobby for policy. His article was an antidote for my lurking doubt, a manifesto for evenhanded writing! But still, a question lingered: Did Drew adhere to these guidelines, or was it just rhetoric? Drew surely held strong opinions. But he appeared to follow this prescribed approach. You can see it in his writing.

Drew's Writing

Drew's policy writing was methodologically sound. He mapped out issues and examined them from all corners. His rigorous analysis of issues is evident even in his response to an unwelcome nomination he received from a presidential committee in 1988 as a "Distinguished Handicapped American." (Ultimately, Drew accepted the award but kept it in a drawer.)

... I must be candid in informing you that there are aspects of the award that give me concern. My concerns are so great, in fact, that I would have had substantial reservations in accepting the award if it had been offered to me. I believe it is important that you and the Committee are aware of these concerns.

First, I am concerned with the name of the award. The term "handicapped" is outdated and is no longer acceptable as a general description of the disabled population. It is particularly inappropriate for the Committee's award, in that it implies that the recipient has been unable to overcome the obstacles associated with his or her disability...

Second, I am concerned about the purpose of the award. If its purpose is to recognize the recipient as a role model for persons with disabilities, it is appropriate that the nominees are limited to persons with disabilities... It could be renamed something to the effect of "Disabled Person of the Year." However, it should also be recognized that an award with this title and purpose has a tendency to separate, and thereby possibly alienate, the disabled population from the nondisabled population.

If, on the other hand, the purpose of the award is, as stated, "for personal and professional dedication to building public awareness of the abilities of people with disabilities," nominees should not be limited to persons with disabilities. There are many nondisabled persons who have made substantial contributions to the public awareness of disability.

Scholars also positively weighed in on Drew's rigorous analysis of policy issues during his tenure review at Florida International University, as did a commissioner involved in a supercompetitive selection process for a national fellowship program, the White House Fellowship.

Chapter 13. White House Fellowship

I am not certain when I first heard about the White House Fellowship Program. I probably learned about the program by reading a newspaper article about one of the fellows, although I am not sure about this. Among the notable individuals whose careers were positively impacted by becoming White House Fellows is Colin Powell,[1] secretary of state and former chairman of the Joint Chiefs of Staff. This seemed like pretty good company to me, and it also seemed like a pretty good roadmap to get from where I was in my career to where I wanted to be. I decided at that time that one day I would apply to be a White House Fellow.

The Fellowship Program

The White House Fellowship Program is arguably the best-kept secret in our country today. It is not meant to be a secret, but if everyone knew what a remarkable experience it is, even more exceptional people would apply for it. Despite aggressive efforts to market the program, it has always been a challenge to reach all of the most promising individuals in a variety of fields to take a year off from their careers to serve in the highest level of the federal government.

The program was established in 1965 during the Johnson administration. It was the brainchild of John W. Gardner, then

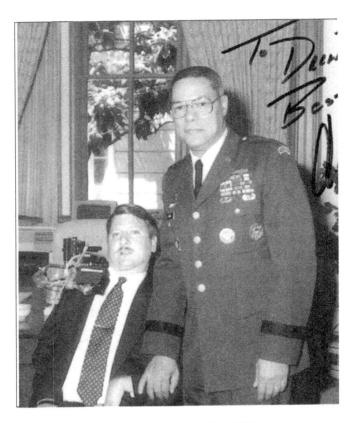

Drew with General Colin Powell at the White House
Fellows office.

president of the Carnegie Corporation, who served as a chief
adviser to President Johnson. The idea was to bring to
Washington, DC, a few individuals from all across the
country who were still fairly early in their chosen careers, but
who had already demonstrated exceptional promise to serve
as leaders. The concept was to take these individuals from
their communities, allow them to experience the federal
government at its highest level for a year, and then to return
them to their communities with an enhanced knowledge and

understanding of how the federal government works (or does not work, for that matter).

The program has three components: the educational program, the work program, and the travel program. The educational program consisted of luncheons two or three times every week at the White House Fellows office with the top leaders in our country. The work program entailed a yearlong assignment as special assistant to a White House official, the vice president, a cabinet member, or other very high-ranking federal officials. The travel program included a major international trip, as well as several domestic trips, in which the fellows toured destinations of interest and met with high-ranking officials in their respective countries or states.

The White House Fellowship Program is arguably the best-kept secret in our country today.

The Application Process

The year I learned about the White House Fellowship Program, I called the fellowship office and requested an application form. I did the same thing for the next three years, never actually applying to the program. Why did I not apply? I really just did not feel that I was ready. Initially, when I first heard about the program, I was working for the federal government and therefore did not qualify to apply. Yet even after I had left DHHS, I did not think the time was right. Every year, I would look at the onerous application form, read about that year's class of fellows, and decide to wait another year. I was determined that, when I finally applied, I was going to be very competitive.

Finally, in 1989, I applied to become a 1990-91 White House Fellow. Completing this application was no small feat.

The application basically had two parts. The first part required you to document virtually everything you had done and everywhere you had been in your life. This was particularly challenging to someone like myself who had already had a couple of careers and who had lived in a variety of places. Simply trying to recall all the addresses and contact people was an enormous endeavor. This information was used by the FBI to conduct an in-depth security check. Those individuals who would be chosen as fellows would have access to some high-security areas, and the federal government did not want to take any chance that enemy spies or other security risks would become White House Fellows.

The second part of the application required the applicant to write two short essays. The first essay was on why the applicant thought that he or she was worthy of this honor and how the applicant thought he or she would benefit from the program. The second essay was actually a policy memorandum to the president of the United States, in which the applicant was required to propose and analyze a specific policy recommendation for the federal government to implement (see Appendix D). The objective of this part was apparently to allow the decision-makers to assess the applicant's analytical and writing skills, as well as the applicant's values, to some extent. Both of the essays were subject to strict word limits, with a warning that essays exceeding the word limit would not be considered.

I wrote my memo to the president on establishing a national personal assistance policy work program to assist people with disabilities in becoming more independent and productive. I had already published fairly extensively on this issue, and therefore I had already thought it through in great detail. The challenge here was to present it in a politically compelling manner within the length requirements imposed by the program. Actually, the biggest challenge was just meeting the length requirement, which was a maximum of 500 words.

I completed my first draft of the presidential memo about seven months before the due date. Much to my dismay, the first draft was slightly too long. In my mind, every word was a gem, and the very thought of eliminating a single word was painful to me. However, the alternative thought of not becoming a White House Fellow due to my unwillingness to compromise on a writing exercise was even more painful. So I started jettisoning full sentences and even a couple of paragraphs. I was very pleased with my ability to transcend my own arrogance, until I realized that, after two months of work, I was still over the word limit.

I spent the next three months in the painful endeavor of eliminating adjectives and adverbs. I spent the month of December figuring out what else to cut; once you have already eliminated all the fat, you must choose between cutting into the muscle or the bone. Somehow, by the due date, I had gotten it down to precisely 471 words. It was one of the best and most tightly written things I have ever authored, though, again, I probably would not have admitted it at the time. Mostly, I was just too emotionally drained to recognize the value of the exercise.

Nowadays, when my students tell me that they cannot comply with the strict page limits I impose on their written assignments, I always tell them this story. The moral is that, with the right motivation, whether it be a gun, a grade, or a White House Fellowship, you can comply with virtually any length requirement. Furthermore, it will usually improve your writing.

Regional Finals

Several months later, in March 1990, I received an official-looking letter in the mail. The return address was the President's Commission on White House fellowships. I eagerly asked my personal assistant, Cheryl, who would later be my wife, to open the letter. One of the most frustrating aspects of being a person with quadriplegia is that you often see things that you want to open immediately, but cannot do so until you are able to obtain the needed assistance. Cheryl opened the letter, which said that I had been chosen as a regional finalist in the White House Fellowship Program. This was very good news.

The way this works is that approximately twelve fellows were chosen from approximately 1,000 applicants in eleven regions of the country. I was one of the regional finalists for the mid-Atlantic region, and our interviews were scheduled for April in a hotel in Washington, DC. Fortuitously, this was the city in which I was living at the time, so this arrangement worked out well for me.

Before I discuss the regional interviews, I realize you might be wondering how one gets chosen as a regional finalist for the White House Fellowship Program. I certainly wondered about this for some time, at least until I was engaged in the selection process a couple of years later. Basically, this is largely a peer review process, whereby former White House Fellows assess the qualifications of potential White House Fellows. Actually, the process is somewhat more complicated than this, in that trained government employees also review the applications, but they do so from more of a technical security perspective.

The former fellows review the applications based upon the primary criterion of future leadership potential; the theory here, I suppose, is that it takes one to know one. Having participated in the peer review process a couple of times, I know the easy part is eliminating the 60 percent or so who were clearly not at the top. The much harder part, of course, is selecting the relatively few individuals who are chosen to be interviewed in the regional finals. At that point, the people are so competitive that choosing the best people is extremely difficult.

The twelve individuals who were selected as regional finalists with me that year were all exceptional people. The good news about this from the program's perspective is that, no matter who is chosen from that point on, the program will be well represented. The bad news about it, from the regional finalists' perspective, is that a single misstep during the regional finals can be fatal, due to the level of competition. Only three regional finalists from each region would be selected as national finalists.

The regional judges are a group of distinguished members of the community, many of whom have national reputations. For example, one of our regional judges was a famous TV news anchorperson, Carole Simpson. I believe there were nine judges in our region all together, and they divided themselves into three groups of three for purposes of interviewing us. Therefore, each of the regional finalists would receive three interviews, and each of the judges would have an opportunity to interview each of the regional finalists.

Although all of the regional judges deserve specific acknowledgment, I will mention only one other judge by name here, because he stood head and shoulders above the rest. I must admit that I had never heard of retired Major General Bernard Loeffke before that day. That is primarily because my knowledge of military affairs is very limited. However, that was not the case of some of my competitors, who informed me that he was a highly decorated soldier in

Vietnam, who in several instances proved himself a true hero, which is a term I do not use lightly. He is a former White House Fellow who also at one time served as the director of the fellowship program. It was clear to me, from the outset, that his views would be very influential, if not pivotal.

For this reason, I was pleased that my first interview was with the panel that General Loeffke chaired. I figured that if he was going to be the key vote, it would be best to be interviewed by him early in what was going to be a long day. I rolled into the designated interview room, pleased that my wheelchair did not bump into any walls in the process. This is not to suggest that I am generally a reckless driver in my chin-controlled, motorized wheelchair. In fact, people often tell me what a good driver I am, to which I always respond, slightly sarcastically, "I practice all the time." However, in this particular setting, you wanted to be absolutely certain that you did not run into anything or anyone, which could raise concerns that the president or his key officials might be in danger in my presence.

These thoughts lead me to some other related thoughts I was having before my first interview. I was wondering, as I often wonder, how my disability would play to this particular audience. I always assume, unfortunately, that it is going to have some effect, though I seldom can predict what it will be. Some people have very deep-seated prejudices against people with disabilities, which they simply cannot overcome even if they recognize on an intellectual basis that these are unjustified. If any of the judges had this problem, I could be out of luck. Conversely, some people bend over backward for people with disabilities and give them more than they deserve. In this sense, we are similar to people of other minorities. I just wanted to be treated on an equal basis with my competitors; that is all I have ever wanted.

In any event, I entered the interview room without incident and I situated myself in the middle of the room so that I could maintain good eye contact with each of the judges. Upon entering, I greeted them with a friendly "good morning." They returned the greeting, which were the last words I heard from them for what seemed like a fairly long period of time. All three judges were looking down at their files, apparently thumbing through the numerous pages of my application, including my policy memorandum.

I had a sense that the other two judges were waiting for General Loeffke to take the lead. He was a striking-looking man with a shaved head and the serious but relaxed demeanor of a person who had achieved great things in his life. He looked impeccable in his uniform, and although he seemed a relatively young man, possibly in his fifties, he also had an almost ageless quality about him. After glancing through my application for some time, he looked up and stared at me for what seemed to be another short eternity. Finally, the following words came out of his mouth: "I see you as a leader…"

I honestly cannot remember the words that followed this. These words were simply the premise to some question that he wanted me to answer. I still am not certain why he used these words. Maybe all of the candidates received this introduction, though I did not have this impression. Maybe he was impressed with the schools I had attended or the number of my publications at the relatively young age of thirty-four. Or maybe he was impressed that I had achieved whatever I had achieved despite a certain amount of adversity. What I do remember is that I thought this was a very nice way to start an interview. As long as I did not say anything remarkably stupid, I had a fairly good chance of being selected as one of the three finalists.

I do remember one very tough question that General Loeffke posed to me. It was his very last question, and I was concerned that my answer may not have been adequate. He said, "You're aware that the purpose of this program is to educate our future leaders about our federal government; you are already a Washington insider, so why should we give you this opportunity, rather than someone who is not politically sophisticated?" My response was basically that just living in Washington, DC, does not necessarily make you either an insider or politically sophisticated. As the words came out, I thought that this response may have come across as somewhat disingenuous, in that I fancied myself as being fairly politically sophisticated. However, in the next few years, I would learn that my response was actually accurate.

I must have done OK, because I received another official letter a couple of weeks later inviting me to participate in the final selection weekend in May.

The National Finals

There is no real way to prepare for the White House Fellowship selection weekend. This entails three days of being interviewed by, eating with, socializing with, and otherwise interacting with members of the White House Fellowship Commission, about fifteen highly successful individuals who are appointed by the president of the United States. If you have flaws, whether they be personal or intellectual or other, they were going to find them. During the selection weekend, the commission included Roger Porter, a professor at Harvard's Kennedy School of Government who was on leave while serving as a chief domestic policy adviser to the first President Bush. Like General Loeffke at the regional finals level, Porter seemed to be a key player. He was also a former White House Fellow and had been appointed to the commission several years earlier.

When I said that you did not prepare for this competition, I meant that you really cannot change yourself at the last minute to conform to what you believe the judges want. You are basically what you are at that point in time, and you must work with whatever skills and accomplishments you have attained at that time. There are, however, some things that you can do, in a sense, to prepare yourself for the competition. One thing you can do is what I did: wait to apply until you feel that you will be a strong competitor. When I finally applied, after waiting several years, I had concluded that I had a real chance of getting this. Another thing you can do is to seek out a mentor, that is, a former White House Fellow who can tell you basically what to expect. There is nothing against the rules in doing this, and most of the finalists had a mentor, or at least some former fellow, with whom they had talked. I was fortunate in that I did not have to seek out a mentor; a mentor sought me out.

Kien Pham is a former White House Fellow and one of the most interesting fellows in the history of the program. He arrived in this country when he was young boy, as a refugee from Vietnam. I remember one time we were talking about our preferred types of vacation, and I suggested that he might enjoy taking a cruise sometime. He immediately put on a somewhat disturbed face and said, "I am a boat person." I suppose that he was not eager for any further water travel. In any event, prior to this little incident (which was actually all in good humor), Kien had generously contacted me and offered to give me some background on the selection weekend. This is how we met and how I got to know him. We had him over to my apartment in Southwest Washington, DC, and he told me what to expect, including a little about the commissioners who would be judging me. His advice was that I should be myself, which is basically what I was going to do anyway. Still, his strong support and interest meant a lot to me. Perhaps most helpful, he confirmed that I would be very competitive.

One thing I may have neglected to mention is that Kien is blind. At the time, he still had some of his sight, but it was diminishing rapidly as a result of a progressive eye disease. I consider myself fortunate, in that my disability occurred at one moment in time and is not progressive in nature. Having a progressive disease would be very challenging, and I truly admire those who are able to handle the transition as well as Kien has. Why he contacted me initially, I do not know. Maybe it was because he identified with me as a person with a disability. I am sure that it also had do with his general desire to help another person, irrespective of disability. Whatever the reason, I very much appreciated it.

Several years later, I passed the favor on. Upon learning about a White House Fellows finalist in Miami, I contacted her and made the same offer that Kien had made to me. We had her to our house for dinner, and I prepared her for the experience, to the extent that one can be prepared for the selection weekend.

The Selection Process

The selection weekend is a little bit of a blur in my memory. This is in part because it was so intense and continuous, and consequently the different components tended to blur together like a surreal collage. Virtually every minute of the three days was scheduled with interviews, meals, social events, and opportunities for recreation, with the exception of several hours that were allocated to sleep.

All together, there were about thirty candidates for between twelve and nineteen fellowship positions. The commissioners had the authority to determine the number of fellowships in any particular year. I believe that several factors go into this determination. There is a trade-off between having a lot of fellows, which is logistically challenging to the program due to the need to place every fellow in a high-ranking position, as well as scheduling issues, and having too few fellows, which limits the opportunity to increase the number of fellows who are providing leadership in their communities. Ultimately, I believe that the commissioners attempt to choose as many fellows as they believe have true leadership potential; conversely, they attempt to ensure that nobody who is selected could be an embarrassment to the program.

Although I did not have an opportunity to really get to know my competitors, in part because it was more important to get to know the judges than the competitors in this situation, I did assess that they were individuals of very high caliber generally. This leads me to an important point. Not being selected as a White House Fellow during the selection weekend is by no means an indicator of failure in life. To the contrary, there is a fairly long list of people who were not selected as fellows, either in the regional or national finals, and who went on to have excellent careers. For example, there was one Hispanic individual who I liked very much who was not accepted into the program, but who is currently regarded as one of the best county commissioners in Miami-Dade County, where I live. I believe that having been selected as a finalist is a strong predictor of success, whether or not you are chosen. Still, this is little consolation for those who are not selected. I certainly would have been disappointed if I were not chosen, particularly after all that effort. I know one individual who made it all the way to the finals without being chosen.

However, I'm getting ahead of myself here. First, I should talk about what occurred during the selection weekend, to the extent that I can recall it. My experience was somewhat different from that of my competitors. They were all there alone; they were not allowed to bring along spouses, significant others, or anyone else. Due to my disability, I had to be accompanied by my personal assistant, who was Cheryl at the time. Generally, I would have regarded the need to have my personal assistant with me in this process as a disadvantage. However, Cheryl has a wonderful and supportive personality and it was good to have her along. Still, having another person in the equation did increase the complexity of the situation. Cheryl was concerned that she would do something wrong, such as use the wrong silverware, which would be held against me. I assured her that, if anyone was going to screw this up, it was going to be me.

Fortunately, I did not. However, Cheryl and I did witness a couple of my competitors self-destruct before our very eyes. At the very first dinner together on Friday night, with all of the competitors and commissioners seated together in a large dining room, one guy stood up and proceeded to make a constructive criticism of the selection process. Remember that I said that one of the primary objectives of the commissioners was to weed out anyone who would be an embarrassment to the program. I am not sure what this guy had in mind when he stood up. I cannot remember the particular criticism that he presented. However, that did not really matter, because he was one competitor who was no longer in the competition. Maybe he thought that this strategy would somehow distinguish him from the rest of us. If that was the theory, it worked, but not exactly as he intended. It created the perception, and the risk, that this individual might have a similar outburst at a state dinner or other important function.

Another competitor—this time, a woman—also self-destructed, though not as rapidly. Every time this individual showed up for an interview, meal, social function, or whatever, she had a different hairdo and a different outfit. One minute her hair was up, the next minute her hair was down, and then it was on the side (french braids, a ponytail, a bun, and numerous other styles whose names I do not even know). Just when I thought that I could identify who she was, she changed her look entirely. I am not sure what type of fashion statement, or other type of statement, she was trying to make. However, if her objective was to be selected as a White House Fellow, this was another bad strategy for doing so. Her impressive performance as a quick-change artist at best conveyed that she had misplaced priorities, and at worst conveyed that she was a little crazy, or at least not as stable as one would like a high-ranking government official to be. What she was offering was not what the commissioners were looking for, and she was soon out of the competition.

Fortunately, I did not make any major mistakes. Generally, I thought that I was doing very well in the interviews. I have always done well in job interviews, and this was in some ways the ultimate job interview. The interviews seemed absolutely endless to me. I actually enjoyed the idea of being scrutinized by such an accomplished group of people, and I liked participating in the first two sets of the interviews. However, after a while, the questions started to repeat themselves, and the interviews started running together in my own mind. This itself was probably a valuable part of the selection process, in that you are more likely to reveal your shortcomings when you are exhausted and responding to the same questions over and over again. Apparently, any flaws that I may have revealed were not serious enough to prevent my selection.

I did have one minor misstep in the process. During one meal toward the beginning of the weekend, Cheryl and I were seated at the same table with Roger Porter. I saw this as a great opportunity to have a policy discussion with one of the top domestic policy people in this country. However, I may have been trying a little too hard to impress him. The conversation was going very well until at one point I drew some conclusions about some arcane issue concerning health care policy, and he looked at me as if I had a mild intellectual disability. I must have said something stupid, but to this day I do not know what it was. In any event, it served me right for trying too hard to impress him, and thereby violating Kien's good advice—to be myself.

With that minor exception, everything went very well for me during the selection weekend. I had the sense, about halfway through it, that I had a chance of being selected. During one of the interviews, one of the commissioners stated to me that my policy memo was the best that he had read in approximately ten years serving on the commission. The selection weekend concluded in the early afternoon on Sunday, the third day of the finals. Two days later, I was informed that I had been selected as a member of the White House Fellows class of 1990-91.

My Fellow Fellows

I later learned that I was one of twelve fellows selected that year. This was a very small White House Fellows class. I was pleased about this, in that it made the program more intimate and gave us plenty of opportunities to get to know one another well. This was a truly remarkable group of people.

The White House Fellowship staff, other than the fellows, their principals, and the commissioners, was absolutely key to its success. The staff ensures that everything goes absolutely as smoothly as possible, including the selection process, the assignment process, the luncheons, and the trips. This involved an enormous amount of planning and ongoing implementation. Consequently, it requires the organizational skills of very capable administrators. Fortunately, we had two very capable individuals at the helm during our fellowship year. Interestingly, they were about as different as two administrators could be. Although they did not always get along with each other very well, and each would probably ideally have liked to get rid of the other, their combination of strengths guaranteed us a very successful year.

However, before I describe the players, it is important to describe the environment in which they worked. The White House Fellows Program is based on the ground floor of an old building at 712 Jackson Place, across Pennsylvania Avenue from the White House and also across the street from Lafayette Square. The building is also very close to the famous Blair House, where important dignitaries visiting the White House stay. Accordingly, the program's location is considered prime real estate, and other federal agencies have often tried unsuccessfully to steal it away. At this point in time, there are enough former fellows of both political parties who are influential enough to ward off such attempts.

Fortunately for me, the program resided in the first floor of that old building, and there was even a long ramp to the back door of the building. I do not know the history behind that ramp, but I was glad it was there. The ramp took me into a hallway with pictures of every class of White House

Fellows, one of which included a young lady in a wheelchair. She appeared to have paraplegia, and I may well owe her a debt of gratitude for the ramp. I believe that I had the most substantial mobility impairment of any fellow in the history of the program.

Once you passed a hallway, you entered into a large room with a long table in the middle. There was a divider in the middle of the room, but it was generally left open, making for a very large space. On either side of the room was a desk, one for the director and other for the associate director. This is where Marcy and Phyllis worked, facing each other all the time. Toward the middle of the year, they started closing the partition in the middle of the room so that they did not have to look at each other. Both were political appointees, and each probably had powerful defenders in the administration, so neither could get rid of the other.

Marcy was something of a wild woman. Typically, when you entered the fellowship office, you would see Marcy with her legs up on her desk, a cigarette in one hand and the telephone in the other. She was a disciple of Ed Rollins, one of the most renowned and respected Republican strategists. Marcy had a very informal style, which suited me fine. There are a thousand Marcy stories, which could be the subject of another book. However, one of my favorites pertains to a conversation we had early in the fellowship year. I was looking at the office pictures of her with several Republican presidents and other officials. I asked her, "Marcy, is that your wall of famous people who have known you?" Her response: "Not in the biblical sense." I thought that this was one of the most clever retorts I had ever heard, and it immediately created a graphic image of Marcy and Dick Nixon together biblically, so to speak. Although Marcy is an attractive woman, this was still not a pretty picture.

As wild as Marcy came across, Phyllis seemed the exact opposite. She was very reserved and had a refined English accent. English accents generally do not do too much for me, in that they often come across as somewhat arrogant and superior, but this was definitely not the case with Phyllis. She was always charming and endearing, as was Marcy, but in a very different way. Phyllis always had her hair up in a bun; I could not imagine Marcy in that hairdo. Both women dressed very well, but very differently. Their different tastes in attire reflected their different personalities and styles; Marcy would occasionally wear sneakers with her dress, while I do not recall Phyllis ever doing this. Phyllis could hardly have been more proper and formal.

Marcy and Phyllis were truly an odd couple. Somehow, probably as a result of their strong commitment to the fellows, they made an excellent management team, ensuring an excellent fellowship experience for us.

A Difficult Decision

At the very beginning of the fellowship year, or possibly before the year started, it became apparent to me that I had to make a pivotal and somewhat difficult decision. At the time, I considered myself to be, and was registered as, an independent politically. In fact, I had a certain amount of contempt for both of the major political parties, as I still do and as many other Americans do as well. In addition, being an independent was useful to me professionally, in that I was a policy analyst and researcher, and I did not want to be influenced by, or even accused of being influenced by, partisan politics. Now I was about to change careers, working in a Republican administration, and I needed to decide whether to choose sides.

Actually, I really did not have to choose sides. The White House Fellowship Program is explicitly a nonpartisan program. You can be a member of any party, or no party, and be selected as a White House Fellow. Politics is not part of the process, or at least it is not supposed to be. Almost everything in Washington is political, and the commissioners are presidential appointees; therefore, it is altogether possible that partisan politics raises its ugly head in subtle ways in the selection process, but I do not believe this happens often or overtly. Our fellows class is a case in point. We could not have been more diverse politically, ranging from very conservative Republicans to very liberal Democrats and one who even bordered on some socialist ideologies. Somehow, we were all selected, so there must be some validity to the nonpartisan thing.

Consequently, although I think I did not have to choose sides politically, doing so would be a valuable thing to do. In Washington, there is a general mentality that if you are not with us, you are against us. In serving in a Republican administration, it would be helpful not to be viewed as part of the enemy. The question was whether I could live with declaring myself as a Republican. Years later, I saw an interview of one of my favorite politicians, former Republican Senate leader Bob Dole, talking about how he decided to become a Republican.

Dole had recently completed his medical rehabilitation after returning from World War II as a war hero with one paralyzed arm, and he decided to pursue a political career. In determining his party affiliation, he went to the Kansas courthouse in which he would have to register his candidacy and asked which party had more supporters. According to Dole, that is how he decided to become a Republican. I am sure that there was more to it than that, and you never know for certain whether he was being facetious, because he has a great sense of humor, but I have a sense that there was a strong element of truth in his statement.

My decision to become a Republican was not quite as politically expedient, though I imagine that it could be perceived as such. I had already been leaning Republican for some time, largely as a result of my disgust with the Carter administration and the general perception at the time that the Republican Party stood for fiscal responsibility. Although it no longer is, I believe that in 1990 the Republican Party actually was more fiscally responsible than the Democratic Party. Still, I did not like the rhetoric coming out of the Reagan administration, and I was not ready to become a Republican until the "kinder and gentler" George Bush Sr. administration. Fortunately, that was when I was selected a fellow.

Later, I will discuss my politics in greater depth, because they are an important part of me (see Appendix E), but for now suffice it to say that my decision to join the Republican Party during my fellowship year was not a major political shift for me. I think the same is true of Bob Dole when he joined the party initially. People with views such as ours, who are often labeled "moderates," can find a home in either major party, if that is what they want.

The Assignment Process

Immediately after the announcement of the 1990-91 White House Fellows, the assignment process began. This was the process by which our work assignment for the year was determined. Basically, each fellow developed a list of federal departments, agencies, and White House offices for which he or she wished to be considered. At the same time, cabinet officers and White House officials were given a list and description of the twelve fellows and could request the opportunity to interview specific fellows.

I developed the idea that I wanted to work in the White House. I suppose that I developed this notion in part because I thought that this may have been the one opportunity in my life to work there, and I generally do not forgo opportunities of a lifetime. In particular, I wanted to work for Roger Porter as a staff member in the White House Office of Domestic Policy. This was a coveted assignment, in part because Porter was a former fellow and a commissioner and consequently had a strong interest in making the fellow's experience as good as possible. Because I wanted this job so much, I put blinders on and did not consider other options.

While I was waiting for Porter to make his decision, and waiting and waiting, the White House Fellows program received an interesting call. Apparently, the attorney general of the United States, Richard Thornburgh, was very interested in bringing me on board. Although I was certainly flattered, I really did not know why he would be interested in me. I will discuss later why this assignment actually made a lot of sense and the Justice Department was really the best place I could be. This experience taught me that you do not always know what is best for you, and you should sometimes heed the advice of those who are wiser than you. Marcy told me from the outset that this was a great assignment. Still, I wanted to wait for Porter's decision, and fortunately Thornburgh understood. I am now somewhat embarrassed that I kept the attorney general of United States waiting for what seemed to be months, but was actually weeks.

Finally, Porter made his decision. He chose Rob, the entrepreneur. By that time, I was just pleased that he had made a decision, so that I could tell the attorney general that I was honored to accept his offer to be his special assistant that

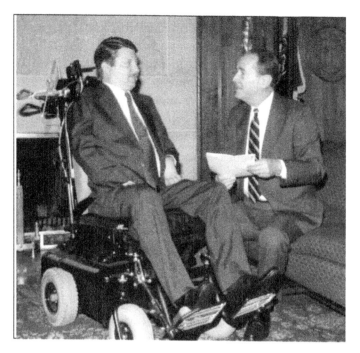

Drew meeting with Attorney General Dick Thornburgh at the Department of Justice.

year. I later learned that Porter's decision took so long in part because there was an ongoing debate within his office as to whether they would choose Rob or me. Apparently, there was a division among his staff as to who would be most useful to them that year. This was important, because White House offices have limited staffers compared with departments, and every staff member is needed to make a contribution. Some of the staff members thought that I would be more helpful because they anticipated health care policy would be a big issue that year.

Ultimately, Porter decided that Rob's business background would be most useful to him, and he selected

Rob. I thought it was a good decision at the time, and I continue to think so. Rob is a very smart guy and is very capable. A couple of the staff members were a little dismayed when Porter announced that one of the reasons he chose Rob was that he was impressed with the way in which Rob attempted to return his shots when they were playing tennis together during the selection weekend. Their point, of course, was that if assertiveness and effort on the tennis court was one of the criteria for selection, I really did not have a fair shot. Although I appreciated their show of support, I really did not think the tennis game made the difference, particularly because I may have said something that did not impress him during the competition. In any event, both Rob and I got excellent placements, and we were both happy.

The Fellowship Year

My year as a White House fellow was truly remarkable and would require another full book. However, I will try to convey the essence of the three components of the experience here.

The Educational Program

Two or three times a week, all the fellows would sit around the big table at the fellowship office to have lunch with some notable individual, such as a cabinet officer, Supreme Court justice, media personality, or other renowned individual. Guests would be introduced by one of the fellows and then would speak for as long as they wanted. After their presentation, we would go around the table and ask the speaker any questions that were on our minds. Actually, we were not limited to questions, and we could make any comments or remarks that we wanted.

The one strict rule concerning these luncheons is that everything said is off the record, and we could not even take notes. The purpose of this rule was to encourage complete candor, and it was a good idea. Of course, there is really no such thing as complete candor in Washington, DC, but the fellowship program achieved about as much candor as could be hoped for in such a program, and we heard some interesting things that you would not read in the newspaper.

When I said that all the fellows attended these luncheons, this was not completely accurate. All the fellows who did not have overriding work obligations attended the luncheons. This meant that those fellows who had "real jobs," such as Rob at the White House, often had to opt out of some of the luncheons due to a pressing obligation. Those at the White House, in particular, had to opt out fairly frequently because the White House is often in crisis mode or semicrisis mode, and every body and mind is needed.

In referring to these as "real jobs," I do not mean to suggest that others like myself had jobs that were somehow not real. We were expected to be at work on time every day, and to fulfill our responsibilities, some of which were substantial. However, we generally had the flexibility to participate in almost all of the fellowship activities. Attorney General Thornburgh was particularly good to me, in that he recognized that this fellowship was a once-in-a-lifetime educational opportunity, and I was able to attend almost everything. I really appreciate this, in that I enjoyed the luncheons very much. The last thing I wanted was a "real job" that would restrict me too much. The Justice Department really was the ideal placement for me.

The speakers that year were truly extraordinary. I will just mention a few here. My three favorites were Colin Powell, David Gergen, and Bob Woodward. Colin Powell is a truly remarkable and honorable human being who should someday be president of the United States. He was born in Harlem, in New York City, and rose to become chairman of the Joint Chiefs of Staff and the secretary of state. I suppose that I identified with the fact that he was a member of a minority from a borough of New York City who became a White House Fellow. At the end of the luncheon, each of the fellows had a picture taken with Powell. In my picture, which is hung in my office, Powell is touching my arm in a supportive manner, almost as if to say that he also felt some type of a bond.

David Gergen is the person in the media whom I respect most. He has had a remarkable career, weaving in and out of Republican administrations, editing *U.S. News & World Report,* and later serving in the Democratic Clinton administration (despite being a Republican). In the Clinton White House, which I believe Gergen served in the first term, when it needed adult supervision desperately, he was treated very poorly because he was a Republican. I felt close to him immediately, and I truly enjoyed meeting him and hearing his political analysis, the most astute in the field.

Bob Woodward is another superb media person. He was very candid and interesting. Although I am not allowed to tell you what he said at the luncheon, I believe that I can say without violating a confidence that he did not tell us the identity of Deep Throat, his anonymous source during the Watergate scandal. I found him very engaging and seemingly eager to contribute to our political education. He also conveyed a sense of integrity, as did Gergen, which is often lacking in the press.

Two of my favorite experiences with the education program pertained to situations in which I had to introduce speakers. I should mention that not all of the luncheons were held at the White House Fellows office; some were held in the offices of the speakers. This was the case with my principal, Richard Thornburgh, and Chief Justice of the United States William Rehnquist. I particularly enjoyed hosting our luncheon at the Justice Department and introducing Thornburgh with great accolades. He had been very good to me, and I wanted to express my appreciation publicly.

Another person I was supposed to introduce was Chief Justice Rehnquist. Our lunch that day was held in the Supreme Court building. I gave the Chief Justice a fairly long introduction, followed by: "...and finally, Mr. Chief Justice, on a personal note, I want to thank you for swearing me in to the California bar back when you were an associate justice. You may recall that we broke the Guinness Book record for the most pictures ever taken at a swearing-in ceremony. I'm not sure whether you remember that." The Chief Justice just nodded his head up and down, as if to say he had still not fully recovered from that experience, which was initiated by wonderful colleagues at DHHS.

The Travel Program

The travel that is part of the White House Fellow program is probably best considered part of the education program. The purpose of these trips was to expand our horizons, and they were not boondoggles (i.e., paid vacations). When we traveled, we were considered representatives of the White House, and we were treated as VIPs. We met with some of the top officials in every country or city we visited. Almost every day was scheduled very tightly with meeting after meeting after meeting.

All together, there were three official fellowship trips: two domestic and one international. The domestic trips were pretty much determined at the outset, although there was some flexibility in determining the details. In New York City, we met with city officials, including Mayor Dinkins. With each of these dignitaries, we had an opportunity to hear their spiel and to respond with questions or comments, much like our luncheons in Washington. I told the mayor that I was very pleased to see that he was wearing a small wheelchair-accessible pin on his lapel. I then asked him whether that meant that they would be starting to make the subway system accessible to wheelchairs by my next visit. He just smiled and went on to the next fellow. I was actually not asking a rhetorical question, but I was not going to press him for an answer. New York City has one of the best subway systems in the world, if you do not mind the smell of urine much, and it is neither fair nor efficient for people who use wheelchairs. I would have presented this perspective to him, but I was expected to be diplomatic. As a public official, you are often not supposed to speak your mind, and I did not care for that aspect of the job.

The California trip was also interesting. We started in Los Angeles, where we met with Mayor Bradley and others. One of the most of fascinating meetings, however, was the luncheon with Police Chief Daryl Gates. Earlier that year, Gates attracted national media attention as the result of abusive police tactics in the famous Rodney King case, in which an African American man was beaten while someone videotaped it. We discussed the beating, the media response, and other issues. The specifics, of course, I cannot present.

The most interesting meeting of all was with former President Ronald Reagan at his private office. This was a year or so before he was diagnosed with Alzheimer's disease, and he seemed strong in mind, body, and spirit. As I may have suggested earlier, I was not a big fan of the Reagan administration. Mostly, I did not care for a lot of their "evil empire" rhetoric, and their policies seemed simpleminded to me. Moreover, I always had the feeling that some of his men were racists. I did not think this of Reagan himself, and I do not believe he had a mean bone in his body. I also did not think he was very smart, and I used to cringe whenever I saw one of his press conferences. However, his prepared speeches were an entirely different thing. I was always prepared not to like what he had to say, and I usually did not like it. However, I did not sit through any of the speeches without having a smile on my face. He had the most remarkable charisma I had ever witnessed, which was somehow transmitted through the television set. I could not dislike him, as much as I would try. I always wondered what it would be like to meet him personally. I had that opportunity in his LA office one day in 1991. He did not disappoint me. He seemed to have a glow about him. I have never met anyone with this much charisma. Even Bill Clinton, whom I met years later and who also has this gift, does not compare. I was prepared to ask Reagan a tough question concerning why the federal debt ballooned on his watch. At the last minute, I decided not to ask the question, in part out of respect for some of my colleagues, the Republican fellows who practically worshipped the man. Mostly, I backed off out of respect for this former president, with whom I disagreed on almost everything.

My greatest political victory in my fellowship year pertained to the international trip. It was a political victory because we, as a group, had to decide where to go. I wanted very much to go to the Far East. Although the other fellows came up with some other options, the final vote was between the Far East and Africa. Ultimately, my preference prevailed, and we went to China, Hong Kong, Japan, and South Korea. Among the highlights of the trip were meeting with top officials of each country, eating at the best restaurants, and visiting such landmarks as the Forbidden City in China and the demilitarized zone (DMZ) in Korea, as well as the shopping district in Hong Kong and a commune in China. At the DMZ, we were told that it was likely that sniper rifles were aimed at us the entire time. Apparently, we were not important enough to kill.

However, the highlight of the trip was the Great Wall of China. This was in part because it really is one of the great man-made wonders of the world. It is about 3,000 miles long (the equivalent of building a very high wall from New York to San Francisco). This is all very impressive, but not as impressive as how I got to the top of it. This was no small feat. In order to get to the top, I had to climb about five flights of stairs. My wheelchair does not climb so well, so I would need to depend on some very strong people. Fortunately, my class of fellows made this a team goal. They were going to get me to the top of the Great Wall if it was the last thing they would do!

I was in my manual (i.e., nonmotorized) wheelchair. I always travel in that chair because I have a theory that the airlines have a demolition crew that they assign to destroy my chair; there is much less damage they can do to a manual wheelchair. It was fortunate that I had the manual chair, because there is no way that we could have gotten the motorized chair up there. First, there were two sets of about fifty steps each. Then there was a cable car that took you to the base of the wall. The thing about the cable car was that the door of each car was only a half inch wider than my chair. In addition, the cable car did not stop, so we had a very limited period of time to get the chair through that door and get out again when we reached the top. Once we got out of the cable car, which creaked as much as our Air China jet shook, there were still two sets of spiral steps to the top of the wall. These steps had just enough turning radius to accommodate my wheelchair. You might be wondering if all of this was worth it. My answer is a definitive yes. Of course, I am really not the one to answer that question, as I was not the one doing the heavy lifting. That credit goes to the male fellows, several of whom are military guys and all of whom are can-do guys. I had no doubt that we were going to make it; my only role was risking my life, and I did not perceive that risk to be very great. Moreover, if I was going down, a lot of other people were going down with me. I believe that if you were to take a poll of all the fellows that they would unanimously agree that it was worth the effort. Everyone seemed proud that we had made it to the top of the wall, which seemed like the top of the world on this most beautiful day. They had helped me achieve one of my dreams, and they did it with a triumphant group effort. I have the picture to prove it.

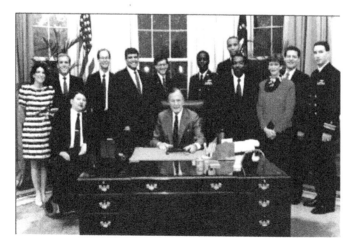

President George H. W. Bush, meeting with the 1990-91 White House Fellows.

The Work Program

Finally, I believe that the most important component of the fellowship year was the work program. Being assigned as a special assistant to a cabinet officer or other high-level federal official is a great honor, privilege, and opportunity. When I say "opportunity," I am referring to the unique opportunity to observe firsthand the leadership style of one of our nation's foremost leaders. Although I am certainly biased, I believe that my principal, Attorney General Thornburgh, was the very best of the best. His reputation was one of several reasons that Marcy had encouraged me to accept the Justice Department assignment.

I owe Marcy a debt of gratitude for her wise counsel, but I owe an even greater debt to my principal, Attorney General Richard Thornburgh, for sticking with me and understanding even when I did not deserve his patience. I had a lifetime's worth of travel and educational experiences that year. I developed friendships and working relationships that have remained important to me until this day, and that I will always cherish. However, working with Thornburgh was the greatest experience in a year of great experiences. I discuss this experience in the next chapter.

Commentary: The Trip to the Great Wall of China
/Mitchell Batavia, Brother/

Drew loved to travel, and the Great Wall of China was one destination on his bucket list. His dream was realized in 1990 with the White House Fellows' help. Ironically, scaling the barrier-ridden wall in China occurred around the same time Drew was drafting the barrier-free ADA regulations in America. At his memorial service, Rob Chess, one of the

White House Fellows, remarked (in a letter) on their memorable ascent:

> The highlight of our fellows year was our trip to China and the Far East. The class was split on whether to go to Africa or Asia, but Drew's vision of Peking duck and hot and sour soup carried the day. One of Drew's life ambitions, of which there were many, was to go to the Great Wall of China. And I don't mean just go, but climb on top of. As you might imagine, China is not the most wheelchair-friendly country. The great emperors, in their all-knowing wisdom, somehow forgot to put in ramps. So after Drew checked out each of the forty-two tacky tourist stands on the walkway below, all the fellows took turns pulling up Drew's wheelchair, one stair at a time, for what must have been enough vertical climb for the sequel to *Into Thin Air*. When we finally reached the top—and all of us except those from the military were suffering from a combination of heat prostration, exhaustion, and muscle lactic acid buildup—Drew was wearing a smile that stretched from Outer Mongolia to the Great China Sea. The Great Wall has finally met its match.

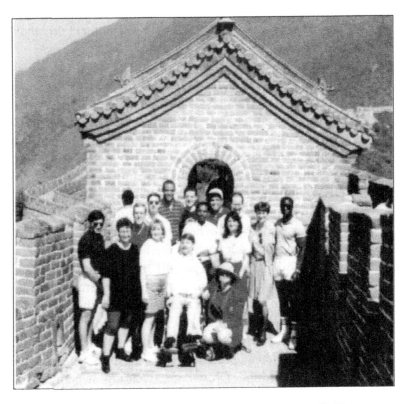

White House Fellows on the Great Wall of China near Beijing.

Chapter 14. The Department of Justice

If you were to have asked me in 1989 as to where I was least likely to work in my lifetime, the US Department of Justice could easily have been on that list. This is, in part, because I was a health care policy guy, and I would have assumed that the Justice Department did not address health policy. I would have been wrong. It would also have been, in part, because I really did not consider myself primarily an attorney. When I went to law school, it was with the intent of becoming a policy analyst. At the Justice Department, I figured that I would be surrounded by lawyers dealing primarily with the courts and judicial policies, which was not all that appealing to me.

It turned out that I really knew almost nothing about the Justice Department. I may be forgiven for this ignorance, because I believe that the vast majority of the American public, including attorneys, knows very little about the Justice Department (or any government department or agency, for that matter). Providing such firsthand, experiential knowledge is precisely what the White House Fellowship Program is about. The US Department of Justice is arguably the most powerful department of the federal government and is involved in almost all aspects of domestic policy in one way or another. Still, health care policy was certainly not its primary responsibility, and it seemed like a strange place for me to be.

How Justice Found Me

Why I was not eager to work at the Justice Department, based on my ignorance of it, is not very difficult to understand. What was much more difficult to understand is why Attorney General Thornburgh wanted me to work for him. I suppose the fact that I was a lawyer, and that I had attended two of the best law schools in the country, was part of the reason he wanted me. However, there were several fellows that year, many who had graduated from top law schools and all of whom were excellent lawyers, such as Jody Greenstone Miller, Sam Brownback, Will Gunn, Kimberly Till, Randall Kehl, and Joseph Samora, and there were plenty of Harvard and Stanford graduates available in the Justice Department generally, so this was no great novelty or attraction.

Another factor was that the Department of Justice was responsible for issuing regulations for implementing the Americans with Disabilities Act (ADA) by July 26, 2001, which was about a year from then. The Justice Department had a strong memory of the last time the government failed to issue disability rights regulations on time, back in 1974, when disability rights activists conducted organized protests in several cities, including a sit-in at the Federal Building in San Francisco. It did not want a repeat of that public relations fiasco.

Moreover, Attorney General Thornburgh was deeply committed personally to the rigorous implementation of the ADA. This commitment was influenced by the fact that he has a son, Peter, who has physical and intellectual disability. Support for disability rights laws tends to be somewhat less politically partisan than other civil rights laws, because disability does not discriminate on the basis of political party; people of both major parties have disabilities, including two of my good friends who are Republicans, Evan Kemp and Justin Dart (both of whom served in the first Bush administration).

One of the reasons that I decided to become a Republican was that George H. W. Bush strongly supported the ADA. I was actually one of the thousands of disability rights advocates who assembled on the White House lawn on a beautiful July 26, 2000, to witness the first President Bush's signing of the ADA. This signing ceremony broke all records in terms of attendance. I regretted that I was not more involved in the enactment of this landmark civil rights legislation. I was involved in research at the time, not legislation, though I did testify at a public hearing held at the National Rehabilitation Hospital, where I worked. Then I learned that the Justice Department would be taking the lead on developing some of the most important regulations for implementing the ADA, the regulations on Title III of the act, which deals with access to places of public accommodation such as banks, hotels, restaurants, and stores. The opportunity to work on these regulations was very attractive to me.

Attorney General Thornburgh

Dick Thornburgh is a remarkable man. He was a two-term governor of Pennsylvania, one of our largest states, continuing a tradition of excellent gubernatorial leadership of that state going back to colonial times. During his second term, his skills were challenged by the accident at the Three Mile Island nuclear reactor, and he proved up to the challenge, avoiding a panic. Thornburgh had earlier served as assistant attorney general in the Justice Department, where he led efforts to prosecute white-collar crime and organized crime. This experience gave him an understanding of the Justice Department that would serve him well when he became attorney general.

Thornburgh was a true public servant. I use this term very carefully, because it is one of the most overused and inappropriately used terms in the English language. Just about everyone in Washington considers himself or herself to be a public servant. If this were actually the case, the public would be in much better shape than it is. In my admittedly cynical view, many of our "public servants" at the highest level are much more concerned with serving themselves or special interests than the broader public interest. Some have made great financial fortunes for themselves and their families while supposedly serving the public, and nobody asks how this is possible. Thornburgh, on the other hand, has served the public well while subordinating his own interests to those of the broader community. Over my year in the department, I developed an enormous admiration for him.

Working for Attorney General Thornburgh had the added benefit of getting to know and becoming a friend of his wonderful wife, Ginny. Ginny married Dick several years after his first wife died in the car accident that also resulted in their son's brain injury, causing his disability. In her efforts to help their son address the challenges of his disability, Ginny became very involved in the disability community. Due to her strong faith in God, she was also involved in many religious causes. When I met her, she was working as the director of the Religion and Disability Program at the National Organization on Disability in Washington, DC. I worked closely with this organization, so I got to know Ginny fairly well. She has become a good friend.

My Relationship with Thornburgh

In suggesting that I had a good relationship with the attorney general, I do not want to suggest that I was by his side at all times. He had several aides who had direct access to him all the time. These were people he had known for a long time, some of whom worked for him when he was governor of Pennsylvania. These individuals were very capable and dedicated to him. Without exception, I liked them very much. The attorney general relied upon them heavily for the amount of staff work necessary to run an enormous federal department. In working with this staff, he had one major rule: no surprises. In other words, staff were expected to keep on top of all issues that affected the office of the attorney general, and he did not want to be surprised by an unexpected question from the press, the White House, or any other entity outside the department. I think this was a very good rule, but it also imposed a lot of pressure on his innermost circle.

I believe that I could have become one of that innermost circle if I had wanted. In a sense, I was a member, in that I interacted with these long-term staffers on a daily basis. Yet, in another sense, I was not a member of that circle, in that I was exempt from the daily responsibilities of the other staffers, which made them subject to the "no surprises" rule. Again, I believe that I could have changed this situation with a single request. It would have required a certain amount of trust on his part, but I believe he would have been willing to take that leap of faith if that is what I wanted. That is really not what I wanted. Some of my fellows wanted that type of responsibility and the relationship that comes with it. For example, Rob Chess had that relationship with Roger Porter at the White House. This made some sense for him, because he was a businessman, and he was going back to being a businessman after that year, and this was his one opportunity to be a real White House staffer. I would have other opportunities to be a "real" staffer, and I cherish the one-time, preferred status I had that year. This raises an important point that I did not mention earlier. If he wanted, the attorney general could have insisted upon my serving as a real staffer. He did not.

Something I did not mention earlier is that I learned very early in the year, before I accepted my assignment, that Dick Thornburgh had actually applied to the White House Fellowship Program in 1963, and he made it to the finals. As I also suggested earlier, the quality of the finalists is so uniformly high that many extremely capable individuals are not selected and go on to remarkable careers. Attorney General Thornburgh is certainly a case in point.

*"The ADA had many fathers,
but Drew, for sure, was its midwife."*

The ADA Regulations
/Mitchell Batavia, Brother/

And as part of Dick Thornburgh's remarkable career, he oversaw the implementation of the Americans with Disabilities Act of 1990. This landmark piece of legislation (modeled after the Civil Rights Act of 1964 that outlawed discrimination based on color, race, sex, religion, or national origin), protected the rights of more than 54 million Americans with disabilities. But the ADA required regulations—and Drew was in the right place at the right time to help write them. While Drew regretted not participating more in the enactment of the law, he contributed when it was time to draft the regulations. As activist Hugh Gallagher wrote of Drew:

The ADA had many fathers, but Drew, for sure, was its midwife. He worked on drafting the language of the act and followed through on drawing the regulations necessary to implement the act. The law means nothing until its regulations are promulgated, and this is what Drew did.

At a fundamental level, the law protects against discriminatory hiring practices simply because of your disability if you were otherwise qualified and could be reasonably accommodated at work (so one can work). It also ensures that individuals with disabilities have access to transportation such as buses and trains (so one can get to work) and access to public spaces like government buildings and new construction (so one can get into work). Even movie theaters were not untouched by the ADA, requiring venues to include closed captioning for people with hearing impairments and audio description for those with vision problems.

Drew drafted the regulations of the ADA that dealt with public accommodations—a fitting opportunity, as he more than most understood the hardship of inaccessibility. Prior to the implementation of the ADA of 1990, traveling in a wheelchair was a nightmare. Cheryl reflected:

Back then, there were no aisle chairs on planes, there were few curb cuts and ramps when you needed them... Patronizing attitudes were rampant, and there was pervasive misunderstanding and discrimination against people with disabilities in places of public accommodation and employment. While I worked for Drew, I became acquainted with the back entrances, service elevators, and kitchens of some of the best establishments in Washington, DC.

Physical barriers could also be found in Cambridge, Massachusetts, particularly around Harvard Square, prior to the ADA. I remember helping Drew move into his Harvard dormitory; some of Drew's fellow law students watched with curiosity as we moved in. They surveyed stair locations in the building and pondered, in sort of an elitist manner, how we would "negotiate" the steps, an odd yet aptly put query. How would we work over, around, or through these barriers?

The restaurant and pub scene around Harvard Square was not much different. We could not enter the vast majority of establishments—some were down a flight of stairs, others were up a flight. You ended up choosing a restaurant based on access rather than entrée.

And the story was the same in New York City. You were lucky if some willing passersby lent a hand to lift the chair over a store's front step. Outdoors, curbs might as well have been cliffs for people riding power wheelchairs. The solution? Traveling in car-riddled roads—a strategy, however, that could prove fatal.

Our mother recalls a summer day in Manhattan with Drew, who was on break from the University of California:

It was a beautiful summer's day, and the family decided to spend the day in New York City. We drove the van down from Yonkers and proceeded to look for an indoor parking garage in the Theater District. We soon learned that raised-roofed vans were not welcome in any of the facilities we explored. We had to go to the other side of the city to park in an open-air parking lot. When we proceeded to walk back to the theater, several avenue blocks away, we found that there were no curb cuts at any of the corners. The only way we could cross the street was to walk down the block and hope to find a driveway to permit us to cross the street and hopefully find one on the other side, permitting us to continue. We were all totally exhausted when we reached the theater. When we presented the tickets, we were told that Drew could not use the ticket because there was no wheelchair accessibility. They of course refunded the money to a very disappointed group of people... On the way back to pick up the van, Drew spotted an ethnic restaurant he wanted to try. Unfortunately, there were two small steps to negotiate at the entrance. We told the manager of our dilemma, and two hearty waiters appeared to help lift the 175-pound load up the stairs. Dinner was delicious, and we wearily made our way back to the van. Drew said, "I love New York."

The New York City subway stations were also substandard for people with disabilities prior to the ADA, and they still aren't too good. In fact, I recall the harrowing experience of getting Drew (and his manual wheelchair) up an escalator in a subway station that lacked elevators. Each time we ascended a step, the moving vertical rise bumped us down a step. It was one of the stupidest situations I ever got us into. In a panic, I lurched backward, using all my body weight, pressing the rubber of the rear wheels into the wall of the step rise, holding my breath, and refusing to budge until we safely ascended to the next floor. I never did that again.

Beyond inaccessibility, Drew also suffered hiring discrimination, being offered far fewer summer internships compared with his fellow students at Harvard in the early 1980s, despite having a similar academic record and likely more charisma. Of course, the practice could not be proved.

All this changed, to a large extent, with the implementation of the ADA. And what did these regulations look like? A portion on public accommodations is included below.[1]

Section 36.201, General

Prohibition of discrimination. No individual shall be discriminated against on the basis of disability in the full and equal enjoyment of the goods, services, facilities, privileges, advantages, or accommodations of any place of public accommodation by any private entity who owns, leases (or leases to), or operates a place of public accommodation.

And "public accommodation" didn't refer only to government offices but included places most people frequent, like bakeries and clothing stores. The regulations went on to say:

Place of public accommodation means a facility, operated by a private entity, whose operations affect commerce and fall within at least one of the following categories—
(1) An inn, hotel, motel, or other place of lodging, except for an establishment located within a building that contains not more than five rooms for rent or hire and that is actually occupied by the proprietor of the establishment as the residence of the proprietor;

(2) A restaurant, bar, or other establishment serving food or drink;

(3) A motion picture house, theater, concert hall, stadium, or other place of exhibition or entertainment;

(4) An auditorium, convention center, lecture hall, or other place of public gathering;

(5) A bakery, grocery store, clothing store, hardware store, shopping center, or other sales or rental establishment;

(6) A laundromat, dry-cleaner, bank, barber shop, beauty shop, travel service, shoe repair service, funeral parlor, gas station, office of an accountant or lawyer, pharmacy, insurance office, professional office of a health care provider, hospital, or other service establishment;

(7) A terminal, depot, or other station used for specified public transportation;

(8) A museum, library, gallery, or other place of public display or collection;

(9) A park, zoo, amusement park, or other place of recreation;

(10) A nursery, elementary, secondary, undergraduate, or postgraduate private school, or other place of education;

(11) A day care center, senior citizen center, homeless shelter, food bank, adoption agency, or other social service center establishment; and

(12) A gymnasium, health spa, bowling alley, golf course, or other place of exercise or recreation.

In 1991, the Department of Justice celebrated the implementation of the ADA in its Great Hall. Drew encouraged the installation of double ramps to better access the Great Hall's stage. And while on stage, Drew introduced the speakers, including Attorney General Thornburgh, who spoke on the implications of the ADA: People with disabilities would no longer be second-class citizens.

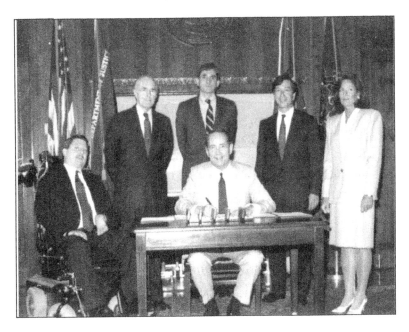

Attorney General Dick Thornburgh signing the Department of Justice's regulations implementing Titles II and III of the ADA, in July 1991. Left to right: Drew, John Dunne (assistant attorney general for civil rights), Tony Schall, John Wodatch, Barbara Drake.

After the ADA regulations were written, Drew personally enforced them. Cheryl and he would scout Washington, DC, neighborhoods in his power chair, noting where curb cuts were needed and issuing complaints to businesses that were inaccessible. These businesses included a bank, camera store, bookstore, cleaners, hair salons, and various food establishments—Chinese, Greek, Middle Eastern, yogurt, and steak house. The couple continued surveillance in Miami Beach following their move to Florida.

Drew also educated the community about hiring people with disabilities. He reached out to elementary school students at Brent Elementary School on Capitol Hill during National Disability Employment Awareness Month to educate kids. Toward the end of the session, after the kids had asked all their questions, Drew had a question for them. "If you were in a position to hire me, would you?" The answer was unanimous: "Yes!"

ADA: Twenty-Five Years Later

Drew's memoir coincides with the twenty-fifth anniversary year celebration of the ADA. During a memorial portion of the celebratory event at the Great Hall, Drew and many others were remembered for their roles in making the ADA a reality.[2]

Over the past quarter century, the ADA has done much to improve access at work and in public places. The Amendments Act in 2008 further clarified the definition of disability so that employers would know when to accommodate. New construction now accommodates individuals with disabilities, and wheelchair users can more easily access city buses, trains, and taxis. However, more enforcement and education are needed. Employment rates for people with disabilities remain low despite ADA efforts to improve access and reduce discriminatory hiring practices.[3]

Chapter 15. A Detail to the White House

/Mitchell Batavia, Brother/

After Drew's work as a White House Fellow at the Department of Justice, he took a position in the White House, serving under President George H. W. Bush, as a senior staffer on the Domestic Policy Council.

President Bush had recently signed the Americans with Disabilities Act of 1990, which was to go into effect in 1992, the same act for which Drew had written the regulations. I'm certain Drew was proud to be connected with a president who put the ADA law on the books. In a recent interview about the ADA's twenty-fifth anniversary, President Bush mentioned that the ADA was among his "proudest achievements."[1]

But the small detail Drew was hired for during that brief stint in the White House had nothing to do with the ADA; it had to do with national health care. Drew elaborated:

Following my fellowship, I served on a detail to the staff of the White House Domestic Policy Council for about six months, attempting to develop a national health insurance proposal for the Bush administration. Despite developing an interesting plan, reactionary elements within the White House ensured that it went nowhere. I have been a long-term advocate of an economically responsible national health insurance plan, and I was convinced that this would be a major issue for the 1992 election. This, in fact, proved to be true, and our failure to propose a credible national health insurance plan did not help the president's prospects for reelection.

Following Drew's stint at the White House, he served a year as research director for disability and rehabilitation policy at ABT Associates, Inc., in Bethesda in 1992, and he worked at the National Council on Disability in 1993. While I do not have much knowledge of the former, I do know something of the latter. He held a top leadership post, executive director, at the National Council on Disability, a presidentially appointed advisory group that recommends policy to Congress and to the president. To give you some idea of this power post, in 1986 his predecessors on the council actually developed the first version of the ADA that was later introduced to Congress.

And Drew fit the mold of a leader. He was well liked, held high standards, and collaborated productively with colleagues on projects. And what was his strategy? Basically, he became familiar with an issue and then respectfully allowed everyone in the room to air their views on it, even if he did not share those views.

I recall visiting Drew in Washington, DC, while he chaired a meeting of the National Council. I watched him advance the agenda as he presided at the head of a room-size table in a packed conference room. It was a side of Drew I had never known. He worked tirelessly, churning out five major government reports on disability policy that had to get published that year. Topics included the ADA watch, minorities with disabilities, access to health services, financing assistive technology, students with disabilities, and an annual report to the president and Congress. However, his work took a toll on his neck muscles, which were overused during the editing process as he pecked out the reports with the use of his mouth stick.

Working in the public sector (and the private sector later) gave Drew the opportunity not just to learn from top leaders, but also to educate them about the injustices imposed on those in the disability community. But Drew was also working on something more personal: marriage.

Chapter 16. Marriage: A Very Good Institution, for an Institution

/Mitchell Batavia, Brother/

Drew became an astute hirer of help, a requirement to stay productive. The alternative was not an option; it's difficult to change the world if you can't get out of bed in the morning. He began hiring attendants while at college. At a minimum, he needed someone to get him out of bed in the morning and back to bed at night and, somewhere in between, to avoid the nemesis that all people with spinal cord lesions face, a skin breakdown over the butt (or, in medical terms, an ischial ulcer).

So after sitting up for ten to fourteen hours, Drew would typically announce, often with urgency, "I've got to get back into bed" or, alternatively, "I've got to get off my butt." The reason was that a skin breakdown, though highly unlikely to occur in a nondisabled person, could easily happen in someone like Drew, who could not shift his weight or sense the warning signs of pain from sitting too long. That could lead to weeks or even months of bed rest in a butt-up position while the raw, ulcerated skin slowly heals. This type of sore, which may start as an innocent red mark on the skin, often belies a more sinister rot, which can morph into a fist-deep wound, florid infection, and take-no-prisoners sepsis. And sepsis, a nefarious blood-borne infection, sometimes leads to death. This made Drew constantly vigilant; he tried to hire attendants who shared the same level of attentiveness.

And Drew hired the gamut, whom he called personal assistants. Some were good, others not so much. The good ones would show up, remember routines, and not kill him via E. coli in his food. Li, a personal assistant of Drew's while he lived in California, was really good. Among other things, he was a professionally trained chef who prepared Drew's favorite meal—French onion soup—on a regular basis. I tried to replicate this dish for Drew but suspected it was never quite as good.

At the other end of the spectrum were the incompetent. The bad ones would miss morning appointments, allow pressure sores to cultivate, undershoot wheelchair targets while getting Drew out of bed, mangle meals that could send him to the emergency room, or simply lack the human virtue of giving a damn. Drew's student hires at UC Berkeley, many of them "street people," fit this category.

And then there was Cheryl. Cheryl fit in the category of terrific. She answered Drew's ad for a personal care attendant in 1984. Eight years older than Drew, she cooked well, but more importantly, she took a robust interest in his well-being. Drew in turn took an interest in her personal development. They were in a sense partners. In fact, it's not uncommon for some relationships like these to end with a ring. Some physicians marry their patients; some professors, their students; and some people with quadriplegia, their personal assistants. This was the case for Cheryl and Drew.

Beyond any romance, Drew needed Cheryl and Cheryl, Drew. She gave him raw honesty, steadfast dependability, wisdom, and multifaceted support, not just in the physical way that a person with quadriplegia requires, but in every other way, so that Drew could live a full life. She carried in her the charm of a Virginian, the poise of a foreign diplomat, the persistence of a marathon runner, and the razor's edge of an editor. She was a teacher, an artist, and a Drew fan.

He gave her the direction to find her professional calling (teaching), a unique window into a life at the cutting edge of national health policy, and what most of us pine for: the need to be needed. Apart from any angst that marriage resembled a shackled institution, as Drew contended, theirs seemed a good fit.

After Cheryl worked with Drew for six years (which, she says, were some of the best years of her life), she completed her teaching degree and moved on with her life, spending a wrenching year teaching first graders in one of the roughest neighborhoods of Southeast DC. Drew had since hired a female personal assistant who had already fulfilled the requirements of being an awful employee. These situations may have served as catalysts for what was soon to be.

Cheryl describes the evening when their lives took a change for the better:

> Drew was also having a difficult time with his new assistant. One night he called me up and asked me to come over to feed him his supper and visit. His new attendant was going to a meeting at her church. My stomach turned flip-flops as I tried to feed Drew the gooey, gray Hamburger Helper his attendant had prepared for him. Then I lay down beside him to watch TV. When I turned him over, I saw it—the beginnings of a pressure sore! I tried to scream, but because I had laryngitis, no sound came out. Drew said he would never forget the look on my face.

It was that night that Drew said, "I need a partner" and asked me to marry him.

We decided that I would move back in and resume his personal care immediately. "But what will your mother think of you living with me if you are no longer working for me?" Drew wondered. Shamelessly, I answered, "If you buy me a big diamond ring, I think she will be OK with it."

That weekend we selected a beautiful vintage diamond ring. I had Drew's wedding ring engraved with something Drew had always told me. He had said he would get married only if "1+1>2."

We had a casual June wedding in our condo's backyard with a jazz ensemble, kids blowing bubbles, beer, barbecue, chocolate cake, and 180 friends and family. I hadn't expected a wedding to mean so much to me, but it was wonderful, and I will never forget it.

What I remember most about their wedding in 1991 was their first dance. Cheryl sat on Drew's lap, and they did wheelchair circles around their guests, who soon joined in. I also recall that some friends, Ruth and Michael Brannon, baked an all-chocolate wedding cake that was decorated with orchids and topped with a bride and a groom in a wheelchair. To fit the toy groom in its wheelchair, its legs had to be broken. This seemed fitting, as one of Drew's legs was broken and in a cast at the time of the festivities.

The wedding morphed into a second day of celebration at Drew and Cheryl's favorite Chinese restaurant, Go-Lo's on H Street in Washington, DC, where they entertained friends and

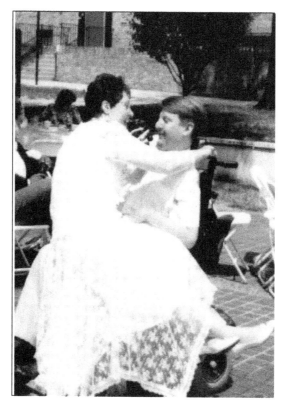

Drew and Cheryl's first dance at their wedding,
at home in Washington, DC.

out-of-town relatives with a formal brunch starring Drew's
favorite, Peking duck. Go-Lo's stood on the site of Surratt's
Boarding House, where in 1865 conspirators plotted to abduct
President Lincoln. After that (the wedding, not the planned
abduction), the newlyweds cruised to Bermuda for their
honeymoon. Drew was a good provider; they enjoyed a total
of nine cruises over the course of their marriage.

In addition to providing, Drew was also a romantic. When
he found out Cheryl had never gone to the ballet, he bought

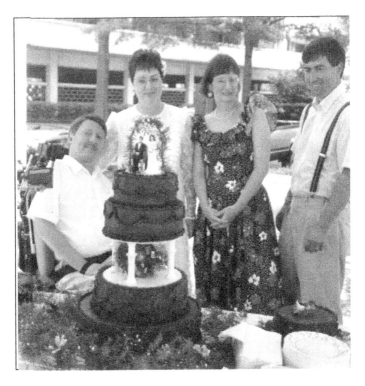

Drew and Cheryl with their friends, Ruth and Michael Brannon, who baked the chocolate wedding cake topped with a bride and a groom in a wheelchair.

season tickets at the Kennedy Center. When he discovered her wish to swim with dolphins, he arranged a surprise family excursion for a dolphin swim. And true to Drew's character, he would regularly bring home surprise gifts such as earrings. I remember walking the street fairs with Drew, something he loved doing, and stuffing little gifts into a pouch on the back of his wheelchair.

On his return home, he would say to Cheryl, "Look in my backpack. I have a little present for you."

Chapter 17. Serving Senator McCain

/Mitchell Batavia, Brother/

Drew started working for US Senator John McCain of Arizona as a legislative assistant in August of 1993, a bit over two years after his tenure as executive director at the National Council on Disability. His office was located off Delaware Avenue in the Russell Senate Office Building, an imposing, trapezoid-shaped edifice faced with marble and limestone and looking at home among the other government buildings. I made one visit to Drew's office during his time there and met several of his fellow staffers, all of whom were bubbly and welcoming. At the time of my visit, the senator was out of town.

As a legislative assistant, Drew focused on what he did best. He worked on domestic economic issues, such as the financing of Medicare and Medicaid and ways to cut government spending. While certainly not sexy topics, that policy could impact millions of citizens. In 1993 Drew wrote on the issue of reducing Medicaid spending by leaving it up to the states to devise their own defensible payment systems. In 1995 he contributed work on taming the ballooning growth in Medicare by reducing government waste, snuffing out fraud, and offering seniors options when choosing medical plans. The idea of giving individuals a choice resonated in all Drew's work, and perhaps McCain's office served as an outlet for this passion.

Drew also wrote five newspaper articles for McCain on health care reform, published in 1993 and 1994. These titles included: "Political Autopsy: Clinton Administration's 'Malpractice' Killed Health Care Reform," "Mitchell Health Bill Just a Clinton Rehash," "Health Reform: A Battle of Opposing Visions," "Alternative Approach: Health Care Reform Should Adhere to Tenets of Free Market," and "Clinton's Cure Worse Than the Disease."

I often wondered what may have lured Drew to McCain's office, other than admiration for the senator and his Republican agenda of less government intrusion. Drew's preface provides clues. McCain spent more than five years as a POW after being shot down in North Vietnam during a 1967 mission. He was isolated, tortured with rope bindings and beatings, and left permanently unable to lift his arms over his head. Perhaps Drew, beyond his loyal political support for McCain, could relate to a man who, like himself, had been confined in some way and still flourished. The two may have shared something in common.

There was something else. It turns out that the senator cosponsored the very Americans with Disabilities Act for which Drew wrote regulations. McCain was not only a strong supporter of the ADA, he was also an ardent advocate of our veterans and a supporter of international disability rights.

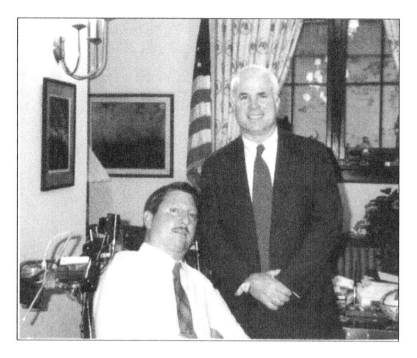

Drew, as legislative assistant, with Senator John McCain.

John McCain wrote a poignant letter, which was read at Drew's memorial service. In it, he writes of a hero:

Drew had to battle every day for the quality of life that many of us take for granted. That he was by misfortune deprived of capabilities that many of us would, were we so deprived, consider essential to a happy life, and yet persevered to make for himself and to help others make for themselves, rich, interesting, accomplished, meaningful lives, dedicated not just to achieving personal happiness but to helping others find their happiness, made Drew a hero to me and to you.

Chapter 18. Semiretirement: Escape to Paradise (Miami Beach)

/Mitchell Batavia, Brother/

After working for McCain for two years, Drew moved to Miami Beach with Cheryl. What drove Drew to move from the politics of Washington, which bustled with action, to the sunshine of Florida, where one retreats for relaxation? Perhaps nostalgia. As children, we used to visit our grandparents in Hallandale Beach during the holiday breaks. The cold winters of DC could have also swayed Drew to move, as snow frustrated wheelchair travels and the cold dampened his mood. Beyond that, individuals with high-level spinal cord injuries like Drew's have thermoregulatory systems that do not adjust terribly well to cold.[1] Florida provided a stable and warmer climate.

Their new home was described as a "unique, 1940 neo-Mediterranean-Deco, five-bedroom abode." Importantly, it was wheelchair friendly. The ranch-style home allowed Drew to cruise independently around most of the rooms and the backyard with only the use of ramps.

Drew installed an automatic door opener on the front door so he could, without help, gain entrance to his home throughout the day. Upon entering, the home opened to a central living room with enough space to make 360-degree wheelchair turns. On the north side of the house, a spacious dining room led to a functional kitchen and a well-appointed (and -attended) family room that accessed the backyard. (That backyard would later sport a premium wooden playground, courtesy of our sister, Donna.) On the south side of the home were the bedrooms, including Drew's master suite with a wheelchair-accessible, roll-in shower. A separate guest suite, which I would use during visits, was situated to the left of the main house entrance.

Drew and Cheryl did experience a few incidents when they first moved into their new digs. On one occasion, an Orthodox Jewish man took it upon himself to walk over to their front door and remove an existing mezuzah (a small parchment scroll whose case can be affixed to the doorframe of a Jewish home as a reminder of faith). Chutzpah! Drew replaced it. Drew had to sue the prior owners of the home for selling the house with a roof that was not up to code. Apparently, they failed to think this through; it's unwise to try to bamboozle a Harvard-trained attorney. And then there were the renovations needed to make the home accessible for Drew, which left them bone-cold during their first Florida winter. But overall, the home was a good fit for Drew and Cheryl. It was, well, paradise.

And what I mean by paradise is that the neighborhood and weather were perfect for Drew. Their home was situated on Prairie Avenue, an idyllic roadway flanked with palm trees and tropical shrubbery, well inland from the Atlantic and west of South Beach. With his power chair, he could independently navigate South Beach (originally a coconut farm and the setting of the film *The Birdcage*), cruise the posh shops and galleries on Lincoln Road, and meander along the historic strip of pastel-colored buildings of the Art Deco

District. What could be bad? The land was flat; the weather, mild; and the culture, humming.

But Drew also needed to find work in this paradise. Although he may have felt semiretired, the reality was somewhat different. He first applied for a teaching position at the University of Miami, but, for whatever reason, he did not get it. However, he did find work as counsel for the law firm McDermott Will & Emery. In a modern high-rise downtown office building, with views overlooking Miami Beach, Drew represented clients in the area of health law. But in order to practice law in Florida, and keep his job, he had to pass the Florida bar.

Cheryl described a cold day when she lent the support Drew needed during the bar exam:

> He was working long hours at McDermott Will & Emery and would come home exhausted, fall into bed, and listen to tapes to prepare for the Florida bar exam. The exam was held at the Fort Lauderdale Convention Center, which was freezing cold. They had assigned someone to write for him who was marginally literate and an atrocious speller, and Drew had to edit and rewrite everything she wrote. About lunchtime, Drew came out with his teeth chattering and said he was not going to complete the exam. I persuaded him to take a lunch break. We walked over to a little diner and ordered breakfast and lots and lots of hot tea. Defrosted and fortified with caffeine and carbs, Drew went back and finished his Florida bar exam. He passed it by only two points.

I would visit Drew on occasion during his lunch breaks at the law firm. We would meet in a nearby public park, where we would talk about his new job. Drew relished his situation, as it allowed him to do pro bono work for disability causes, but he abhorred the life of a corporate lawyer, describing his task of tracking and billing client hours as akin to impaling his eyeballs with ice picks. Law was simply a means to an end for Drew, not to make money but to promote societal change.

Drew also served his community in South Beach. While many view committee work as a whopping waste of time, Drew probably saw how his work on boards could directly impact his community for good. He cochaired the Barrier-Free Environment Committee, served on the Design Review Board in Miami Beach, and was appointed as a board member to the Miami-Dade County Housing Finance Authority. Drew's work on these boards could help shape the look of the neighborhood, especially for those with disabilities.

Beyond local committees and boards, Drew also wrote a column for the *Miami Herald,* penning pieces on such topics as the right to assisted dying, movies for those who are deaf, wheelchair access to beaches, how flat taxes may take more income from people with disabilities, and whether FDR's disability should be visible at his memorial. The common theme, of course, was disability issues.

And while Drew built roots in his community, he was also planting the seeds for a family.

Chapter 19. From Russia with Love

/Mitchell Batavia, Brother/

Drew wanted the "whole experience." He dreamed and lived big but still was not satisfied. He wanted kids.

On the topic of children, Rhonda, our cousin, shares a conversation she had with Drew:

> I approached him one day at the height of his career, while visiting with him in Washington, DC. I inquired whether he would take me up on my offer to write his story. I said to him, "Your life has been so extraordinary. There is so much for you to be proud of." After some reflection, he replied, "No, Rhon, it's not time for that. I really haven't accomplished what I want to." I inquired further, at which point he said, "My goals are to one day get married and have children."

As it turned out, having kids was Drew's final and likely most meaningful mission in life. One hurdle, however, was conceiving, a challenge for individuals with spinal cord injury. And Cheryl, who already was a mom from a previous marriage, was understandably not initially enthusiastic about the notion of having kids. But that all changed with the possibility of adoption, particularly an adoption from the land of Drew's ancestors, Russia. International adoption was particularly attractive, not only because of our roots in Russia (actually Minsk, where our maternal grandmother's family originated), but because Drew was also concerned about a litigious US biological mother later claiming parental rights and taking his children away from him.

As the story goes, when Drew lived in Washington, DC, he attended a luncheon at the Cosmos Club, a private club whose members included luminaries involved in the advancement of the sciences, art, and literature. During the lunch, Deborah McFadden, someone who worked along with Drew in the Bush administration, spoke about an adoption agency she had started in Russia. This intrigued Drew, and after lengthy discussion, he and Cheryl decided to start the international adoption process. Drew's major concern, however, was whether the kids would bond with him, a worry that would have to wait until the children joined their family. Cheryl made the trip alone to the Russian orphanage in the industrial city of Ekaterinburg, 1,000 miles east of Moscow. She spent ten days visiting Joe and Katey before returning to the States with both of them.

Drew described the process of going through the Russian adoption, and the ultimate union and bonding of his new family in Florida:

> ...a high-stakes international scenario was playing out in two of the most impenetrable bureaucracies in the world: post-Cold War Russia and the Clinton administration's Immigration and Naturalization Service (INS). Prior to leaving Washington, we had filled out reams of information and subjected ourselves to the lack of privacy that is reserved under our Constitutional scheme only for

public servants and prospective adoptive parents. Fortunately, we are accustomed to this treatment and breezed through the process with a *maximum* of moaning. Then we were asked to make the most important decision of our lives based on a photograph of Joe and Katey and a one-page medical history for each, which we were informed could be completely accurate or completely inaccurate. (Apparently, Russian officials sometimes manufacture diagnoses to allow children who have not been chosen by Russian parents to be adoptable internationally under Russian law.) Although we could never be sure until they got here, we were able to conclude that they were in good health by demanding a videotape which demonstrated that they were actually superhuman.

Finally, in October '96, all of the necessary bureaucrats at the federal, state, and local levels of each country had signed off on this, and it was time to pick up Joe and Katey. I was then told that I could not be present at the most important occasion of my life, the adoption of my children. (Apparently, the Russians have not yet gotten around to enacting their own special version of the Americans with Disabilities Act.) I hope to have the opportunity to thank them personally for this when we visit Russia, when Joe and Katey are older. In any event, we were given only about two weeks to make the necessary arrangements for Cheryl's trip, because Russian laws change in this area quite frequently, and if we waited any longer, she might have had to spend several months in Siberia, where there is not much to do during the winter (or the other seasons). One of the necessary arrangements was to obtain $9,000 in what we were told must be "crisp, new $100 bills," which were to be paid as "fees" to various Russian officials, who are very picky about the quality of their American currency. Strapping the bills in a money belt to Cheryl's person, to prevent the Russian mafia or other unscrupulous characters during the twenty-four-hour trip from stealing it, this seemed like high international intrigue. Indeed it was, because the stakes could not have been much higher, and there were many ways that this endeavor could have been derailed.

Fortunately, it was not. When my parents and I waited at Miami Airport for over two hours beyond their expected time of arrival, we were concerned that something had gone awry. And then the two most beautiful, intelligent, loving, and mischievous children in all of Eastern Europe emerged from the immigration office screaming, "Papa, Papa" and jumped on the back of my wheelchair.

Drew and Cheryl's home was fully transformed, and life would never be the same again—they were family. And any concern about bonding quickly vanished. Two years after the adoption, Drew described their two amazing kids in a holiday letter:

Joe (alias "Joester," "JoJo," "Crazy Joe," "The Fix-It Boy," and "A Handful"), now eight and a half, is perhaps best described as a Russian-American hybrid of Huckleberry Finn and Dennis the Menace. He recently tried to take a quick spin around the block with my van but fortunately got only a few feet before stopping in the

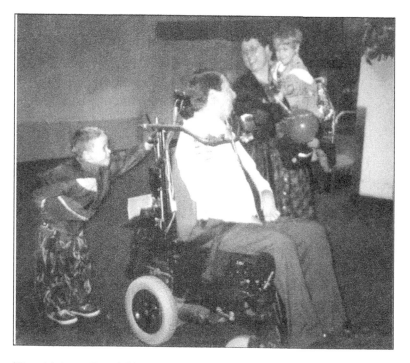

Miami International Airport. Drew meets Joe and Katey for the first time.

driveway. The hint to us was that the driver seat was adjusted to within inches of the steering wheel. On a more positive and less stressful note, Joe fixed my wheelchair on a trip to the Northeast. He has also assembled a cabinet and fixed a TV set. Joe's construction/destruction ratio is rapidly approaching +1, and our main parental objective is ensuring that his talents are used for the good of mankind. He is in second grade and is rapidly learning to read. We are so proud of his remarkable adjustment to this country, though I had not planned to lend him the car keys for at least another eight years.

Katey (alias "The Katester," "Skatey Katey," "Kateybird," "Princess Katerina," "Katey-Pie," "Sweetie," and "Another Handful"), now six and a half, may best be described as Shirley Temple on steroids. Of course, she is not really taking strength-enhancing drugs, but you would not believe the muscles all over her body. And she really packs a punch!!! I learned this the hard way when my far less than perfect body was rendered black and blue when she mistook my bed (and me) for a trampoline during the first month she was with us. It is hard to believe that someone that cute can be that strong. She can lift her thirty-nine-pound body above a pull-up bar four consecutive times, which I believe is off the charts for her age. Skatey Katey is also a wild woman on roller blades, and we are considering the purchase of a new insurance policy specifically for this activity. She is in kindergarten and knows all of the letters and most of the numbers.

Joe and Katey became US citizens that year. In future holiday letters, Joe and Katey took up more and more space on the page, reflecting Drew's increasing obsession with fatherhood:

Both Joe and Katey have continued with their karate and gymnastics. Joe is now a blue belt, which makes him eligible to practice with weapons. Some of these weapons are truly scary things, and I spend a fair amount of effort dodging them for my life when they inadvertently slip out of Joe's hands. It has improved my reflexes. Katey is an orange belt, which makes her less dangerous in the short run, though I can foresee a time in the not distant future when I will be at double jeopardy of being impaled by an Asian instrument of pain infliction.

Cheryl mentioned that both kids loved being read the Dr. Seuss book, *Hop on Pop* and hopping on Papa while he was lying in bed, and "he had the bruises to prove it." She echoed Drew's commitment to his kids and said, "Being a parent was the most important job in his life." Cheryl elaborates:

Drew was born to be a parent. Despite his fears that he might not bond with his adopted children, they quickly became the most important thing in his busy life. Our children hitched rides on his motorized wheelchair to the doctor, to Lincoln Road, and to South Beach. We watched them do gymnastics, karate, ice skating, and roller blading. We took them to concerts, the circus, the beach. We calmly watched as they scaled the bleachers set up for the Orange Bowl parade, various palm trees, and any jungle gym they could find. Drew spent many happy hours watching them do pull-ups and play in the tree house in the gym set generously given to them by Drew's sister, Donna. Later, Drew would take Joe with him to some of the evening classes he taught at Florida International University.

Joe recollects conversations with his dad:

My dad once told me how he became paralyzed at age sixteen. No matter what came along in his life, he never gave up. He always worked on his computer day and night, but when it came to his family, he always dedicated time to us. When he was on the computer, I would walk into his office and ask him, "Would you spend time with me?"

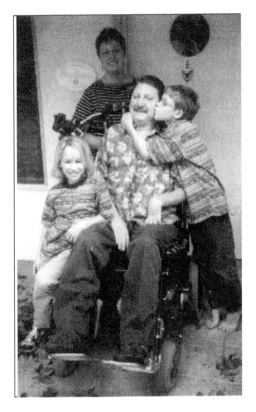

The Batavia family, in front of their home
in Miami Beach in the winter of 1996.

He would tell me, "I'm a little bit busy right now, but as soon as I am done, I promise you, all my undivided attention is yours." Later, he would come to me and ask me, "What do you want to do today?" Sometimes we would go to the beach, Lincoln Road in South Beach, or to the movies. My dad's favorite words were, "What idiot movies do you want to watch?" It would be a joke between him and me, because we would act like kids, giggling and smiling as we watched cartoons. No matter what, Dad knew how to put smiles on our family's faces.

And Katey also recalls memories with her dad:

Dad spent a lot of time with Joe and me. I remember once we were walking on the golf course. My dad ran over our dog Clifford's foot and broke one of his toes. I carried Clifford home, and we took him to the vet. Clifford learned his lesson and never ran in front of Dad's wheels again.

Dad spent a lot of time outside watching us play. He would watch me swing while we listened to music. Sometimes I slept on the floor of Dad's office to keep him company when he was working late on his computer. I always liked to spend time with my dad.

I often wondered if the kids, in addition to fulfilling Drew's wish to be a father, also satisfied Drew's need for an interesting life; it was never dull around the kids. Perhaps he also vicariously enjoyed the children's exuberant mobility. Still, paradise at the Batavias was about to get a bit more joyful.

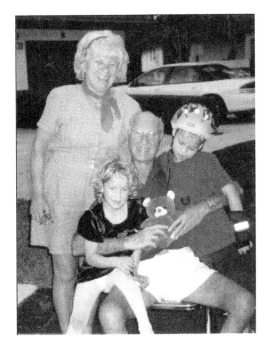

Katey and Joe at Boynton Beach,
Florida,with their grandparents, Renée
and Gabriel.

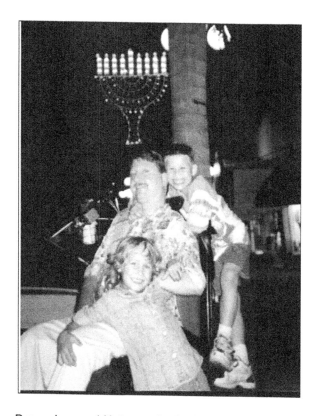

Drew, Joe, and Katey under holiday lights in
Hollywood, Florida.

Chapter 20. Bedlam on the Beach

/Mitchell Batavia, Brother/

After living in Miami Beach for five years, Drew found that there was still a void in the Batavia family's lives. Their house had no name. Drew described their predicament:

> We still did not have a name for our house. It seemed to me that every self-respecting Southern estate deserved a name, and to preserve my delusions of grandeur, our home deserved no less. But what should we call this unique, 1940 neo-Mediterranean-Deco five-bedroom abode of questionable architectural note that would, in a few choice words, adequately convey the essence of its inhabitants and their lifestyle? One Monday, my able assistant James, upon returning from his weekend to two out-of-control children and a house in total disarray, exclaimed, "This is Bedlam!" At that moment, in a fit of inspiration, after many sleepless nights, the name of our residence came to us: "Bedlam on the Beach."

And to counter some of the Bedlam on this beach, Drew declared a "New Joy Initiative" that Cheryl further describes:

He declared that negativity would not be tolerated. It was sort of annoying, but I found that he was right. He never took anything for granted. The New Joy Initiative was a very kind (and effective) way to deal with challenging children and a wife who tends to take it all a little too seriously.

One of the ways joy contributed to their household was the addition of a new family member, Clifford, a lab/chow puppy. Drew described how they came upon this canine addition and the decision to take him home in a holiday letter:

...I received a rare call from Cheryl at her school that went something like this:

Cheryl: "Drew, would you mind at all if I brought home the most adorable puppy that was abandoned and just wandered into my school with two lame legs that may be able to be corrected with extensive veterinary care?"

Drew: "No problem, dear. Just bring him home."

In his letter, Drew elaborated on the dog decision and alluded to some of their previous, less fortunate pets:

Actually, my response did not reflect my complete thought process on this matter. My initial internal response was something like: "Cheryl, have you completely lost your mind?" We had recently received local recognition as the family that had made the greatest use of the Mount Sinai Emergency Room. We had just returned from a "vacation" in which we had blown two tires and lost an axle in between my own set of medical emergencies. And to make things worse, Max I was probably lurking somewhere in the house, and the turtle we had bought Katey to get over the loss of Maxine lasted only three days. I was thinking, during the brief minute I had to respond to Cheryl's life-changing question, that the last thing this family needs is a dog. Then I thought again, how could it make life perceptibly more difficult than it is already? I then uttered the life-changing words, "No problem, dear. Just bring him home."

Drew also commented on the origin of Clifford's name:

Joe named Clifford after the legendary red dog that grew to enormous proportions. True to his name, Clifford was six pounds and twelve inches long when we adopted him at seven weeks, and is now forty pounds and four feet long at five months, and GROWING.

And Cheryl expanded on Clifford's relationship with Drew:

Clifford became the perfect family dog. When he was very small, I lifted him up to lick Drew's cheek and it became Clifford's special job to wash Drew's face every night when I lifted him into bed. Once Drew had a sore on his toe. Medicine wasn't helping, and Clifford kept trying to lick the wound, so finally Drew said, "Let him go ahead and try to heal it." Every day Clifford licked Drew's foot until it healed. After that, he still checked daily to see that Drew's foot was OK.

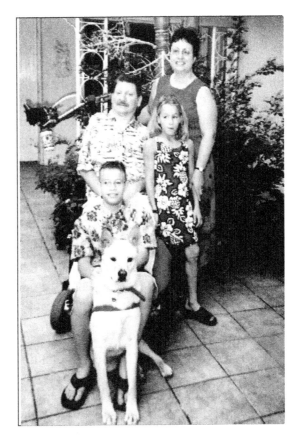

Drew, Cheryl, Katey, Joe, and Clifford at their home, "Bedlam on the Beach."

When Drew died, Clifford, Joe, Katey, and I all slept together in our king-size waterbed that first night. Clifford acted sad and depressed for a month after Drew died and began sleeping at the foot of my bed every night.

Still another tradition of the New Joy Initiative was karaoke, a recreational activity that involves singing out loud to the lyrics of popular songs while the song's music plays in the background. Around that time, Drew and I had published a paper on karaoke as a possible respiratory intervention for persons with spinal cord injuries. Drew described the new tradition in his final holiday letter:

> We must warn you that, as part of the New Joy Initiative, we have purchased a karaoke machine. This means that if you come to visit us at Bedlam on the Beach, you will be required to sing for your meal. However, please do not be deterred, because we all sing in several different keys, mostly the wrong ones. Still, somehow it always comes out beautiful!

Drew also created fun recreational games for individuals with quadriplegia: his blow dart enterprise. Similar to the game of darts, the blow dart kit came with a pipelike dart gun that one would blow through to shoot a Velcro-tipped dart at a hanging target. The game worked the muscles of respiration and was, well, fun. Cheryl shares a story of Drew selling his toy: He was scheduled to market his toy at a disability conference in Puerto Rico, but he almost missed his flight when airport security suspected a pipe bomb in his luggage.

Chapter 21. The Professor

/Mitchell Batavia, Brother/

Drew joined Florida International University (FIU) as an associate professor in September 1997, after working for two years at the Florida law firm. I started at New York University about one year later, a happy accident, as it drew our two worlds closer. FIU is a large research-active public university known for its diverse student body. What is less well known is that it was built upon the tarmac of a decommissioned airport and is thus fairly flat terrain. It was a good fit for Drew: the grounds accessible, the commute doable. Pun intended: Drew took off. He became a professor.

He worked primarily in North Miami's Biscayne campus. His office consisted of a simple space with a computer and reading stand elevated on mammoth tables, high enough to accommodate his power chair and knees below. On the wall hung a print of Don Quixote mounted on a wheelchair and brandishing a spear, a constant reminder of his life's mission.

And Drew's office was a model for the ADA: inexpensive accommodations leading to behemoth productivity. He was staggeringly productive in academia despite his disability, deftly tapped away at his keyboard using a mouth stick at a rate of twenty-five words a minute, a rate that surpassed many who use ten fingers. Unfortunately, he destroyed his neck muscles through overuse while cranking out papers when he served as executive director at the National Council on Disability. Now, as professor, he would rely on voice-activated dictating software to get his papers out.

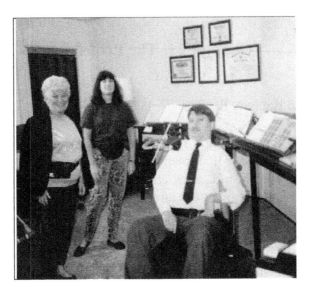

Drew's typical office setup, with elevated tables, reading stands, and a computer. Drew with mother, Renée, and sister, Donna.

The only annoying thing Drew had to contend with in his new office were mischievous pigeons outside his window:

These pigeons seem to be constantly engaged in the act of procreation, which they do not conduct quietly in the privacy of their nest, but rather in a wild, frenetic ritual that involves loud, incessant coooing.

And with regard to the office itself, Drew jokingly started to notice an inverse relationship between his career path and size of his digs:

Admittedly, this office does not have the same ambiance as Eisenhower's old office I once occupied in the Old Executive Office Building, but it does have a certain charm. (Actually, looking in retrospect, I recently realized that, as my career has moved forward, my offices have become progressively less grandiose. I have not yet had time to interpret the implications of this insight, but at this moment I am not unduly alarmed by it.)

Drew was happy as a professor. After teaching an evening class, he told me, "I think I'm gaining a following." I understood what he meant; it's gratifying when you feel like you made an impact on students who may one day carry on your legacy. In fact, it's quite an ego inflator to watch your students take notes on what you profess. One can describe Drew's seven courses, which he taught over his five years at FIU, as rigorous. He taught both graduate and undergraduate students, with up to eighty-five students in a class. I recall looking over one of Drew's FIU course syllabi as I was preparing courses at NYU and getting a knot in my stomach. Reading it was a bit unnerving, akin to entering into an ironclad contract: mandatory attendance, grading criteria, memorandum assignments. Nevertheless, students offered strong reviews of this course.

The life of a professor had many perks, one of which was flexibility. It allowed Drew to work from home and teach at night so he didn't have to sit up for long hours at a stretch. This was good for his buttocks, an anti-pressure-sore strategy.

But the flexibility also allowed Drew to have time with his kids, to go to their school events, or to just be there for them.

And while I mentioned that being a professor had perks, going up for tenure was not one of them. In order to remain at FIU, Drew needed tenure, a typically grueling and protracted process whereby the university examines every detail of your scholarly life with an MRI. It is an intellectual marathon on steroids, and it sometimes can feel like running a race barefoot on broken glass with few cheering you on, and even fewer waiting at the finishing line, as you showcase your productivity as a scholar over several years. But before you get too excited about jumping at this "vacation" opportunity, consider that for the next six years of your life you will eat, sleep, and brush your teeth pondering where you are going to publish your next paper while the university holds a metaphorical gun to your head. If you got tenure, you could stay; if not, you were out.

And although going up for tenure is typically an arduous process, I never heard Drew complain. Remarkably, his dean mentioned, he sort of enjoyed it. I found this odd. For me, it was a gorilla on my back. While it is a major milestone that tests your grit as a scholar, your focus becomes so tunneled that you practically need to reacquaint yourself with your family when it's over. And this brings me to an important point: It is infinitely harder to work toward tenure while raising kids; children, though wonderful, are a major distraction. But Drew did it and thrived.

Drew described this experience with tenure in his final holiday letter of 2002:

This is quite a process that they have devised, which entails my putting together a tenure file of all my work over the past twenty years, and subjecting it to the scrutiny of an unbelievable number of committees and officials. I believe that I assembled one of the strongest tenure files my university has ever seen. So far, I have received unanimous support from the two major committees that have considered me and a strong letter of support from my dean, despite the earlier opposition of one of my program colleagues who hates me. University politics can be pretty nasty! As I understand it, the final tenure decision must be signed off by the provost and the president of FIU, Governor Jeb Bush (who is a friend of mine), President George W (who would probably not care for me much), and finally Kofi Annan at the United Nations. [Actually, this is a slight exaggeration, but only slight.] Wish me luck!

Drew achieved tenure and promotion to full professor posthumously. Needless to say, Drew was not able to experience the entire process while alive, although he submitted everything on time. Just the same, I believe he was privy to the news of the tenure decision during his final days in the ICU. In January 2003, his dean called, while massive IVs dripped medication and EKG alarms beeped at Drew's bedside. I recall that Cheryl's cell phone rang, and she held the phone up to Drew's right ear for what felt like three minutes. Later, at the memorial service, the dean spoke on how timely the tenure process was for Drew, as a wonderful means of reflecting on his own life's accomplishments.

And to give you a sense of Drew's scholarly output during his brief forty-five-year life, let's do a bean count. He cranked out sixty-nine refereed journal articles, three books, thirteen book chapters, twenty-three letters to the editor, eighteen newspaper articles, and two book reviews; he served on forty-seven panel presentations; he was awarded thirteen grants and contracts; and he had nine works in progress—a ridiculously rich tenure file by any standard. His curriculum vitae ran for twenty-eight pages, and, incredibly, his papers required little editing prior to publication. His reviews from experts around the country were uniformly exceptional; Drew was deemed a top scholar in his field. But his productivity speaks to a much larger issue, one of human potential. If someone like Drew, who functioned with only about 10 percent of his body, produced such a massive trove of work in such a brief period, think of the unrealized promise in all of us who operate with far more.

If there was any weakness in his file, it was likely his dearth of committee work within the school, an infraction most serious research-intensive universities don't weigh heavily in a tenure application. Instead, Drew worked externally, beyond school fences and in the national spotlight, an effort that brought attention to FIU. And while he could have published more in law journals, his focus was interdisciplinary, bridging the fields of law, health policy, and medicine.

Drew worked more robustly and produced more work than most of his nondisabled counterparts, and I think he was proud of that. Perhaps he felt them lazy. He pushed hard, as if each day was his last, and perhaps he felt them numbered, explaining his furious race to publish. It also didn't hurt that he worked ten to fourteen hours a day and on weekends throughout his postinjury life. The fact that he celebrated each surviving year of his quadriplegia lends support to this sense of urgency. His hard work paid off. Even posthumously, he is cited by other researchers on a regular basis; his ideas live on. And I would laugh at the irony that he'd get more authors citing his work in death than I get while alive! But the reason for this makes sense. He tapped into a fundamental concern of national interest: equality.

The majority of Drew's publications, which were multidisciplinary, focused on establishing a level playing field for people with disabilities, and many are viewed as pioneering works in the field. These areas included: health service financing, particularly medical rehabilitation; Social Security disability reform; the Americans with Disabilities Act; the independent living model for long-term care; and end-of-life issues, such as the right to physician-assisted suicide, which Drew was likely the first to examine from a disability perspective, in a piece published in the *Western Journal of Medicine*.[1] But if you knew Drew only on a personal level, you would still gain a fresh appreciation of his intellectual capacity after a quick read of his papers; he possessed encyclopedic knowledge of policy and a gift for compelling argument. If he didn't woo you with his first argument, he followed up with six others, all with legal and ethical hooks.

There is little doubt that Drew had international reach within the disability community. Geurt Heijkamp of the Fokus Foundation in the Netherlands wrote, in a letter, about Drew:

When I first heard of Drew, I think it was from Philip Mason, one of the prominent members of the Independent Living Movement for people with a physical disability. I was told to meet "the Wizard." I am almost sure that you have read or have seen the trilogy of Tolkien: *The Lord of the Rings*... In that trilogy there is a character called: Gandalf. He is the wise, humorous, and intellectual person in that story and always honest. Drew was the Gandalf in our movement.

When he died, Drew was just finishing *Independent Living*,[2] a book that examined different care models for living with long-term disability in the US, a topic Drew knew something about, having hired and fired dozens of personal assistants over the years. In fact, he had published an article about a decade earlier proposing a national personal assistant service program in the US as an alternative model for long-term care, whereby nonmedical professionals are hired by individuals with disabilities.

In this book he compared three models of care: an informal (family) support model; the traditional medical model, where health care professionals oversee care; and an independent living model, where consumers are the bosses, hire their own nonprofessional help, and direct their own care. Drew fit into the third, consumer, camp although he believed it may not be a good fit for everyone. In finishing the book, he asked me to help him generate charts, so I was somewhat familiar with what he considered was a "never-ending project." Shortly after his death, it was published, as Cheryl and I promised.

One important area that Drew focused on was the obscene cost of health care in the US, something most of us worry about, and he, having a disability, likely worried a bit more.

Although Drew was a health policy and law expert, he was also a patient who was just as perplexed as any of us when opening a piece of mail containing a hospital bill. The following excerpt from Drew's classic *Lancet* article captures his wit on this topic after spending one day in the hospital with a urinary tract infection.[3] Upon returning from a planned family vacation cruise to the western Caribbean, he opened his mail to find an exorbitant hospital bill. The British editor at *Lancet* loved the piece and was anxious to publish it posthumously.

I decided to have a friendly exchange of ideas over this bill with the administrators of the hospital. I chose to start at the bottom, meeting with the billing person at the business office. This person calmly and politely explained to me that I owed the hospital the amount presented in black and white on the last line on the bill that she had diligently sent me. I calmly responded to her that I knew how to read the numbers, and that I was really looking for an explanation as to how they were derived. She made clear at that point that she could not help me understand this, in that such determinations were made well above her pay grade.

I then asked how I could talk with the chief financial officer of the hospital, thinking that I should now shoot for the other end of the administrative spectrum. I further learned that she was a graduate of the very health services administration program in which I teach. I was eager to congratulate her on how much she had learned from our program. Since I do not teach price theory, I have often wondered how administrators set the prices for health care services. I had always assumed that they assign the highest price that they believe they can submit to insurers without laughing out loud—the so-called "straight face test." In billing over $3,000 for my one-day stay, I figured she must be very talented.

Unfortunately, I was told that the chief financial officer was on what I am certain was a well-earned vacation. I was therefore delegated to her assistant, with whom I engaged in the following fascinating conversation:

Me: I appreciate your taking the time to meet with me. I am a health care lawyer and a professor of health law at Florida International University. I was a patient at this hospital last month for one day, and I am not happy with your bill.

Administrator: Hi, I'm a CPA and the assistant to the CFO. I'm sorry to hear that you're unhappy. Let me look at the bill. Good, everything looks in order.

Me: You are aware that this hospital bill is for over $3,100 for a one-day stay? Actually, I was admitted at about 4 p.m. on Thursday and discharged about 11 a.m. on Friday, which is about nineteen hours. That comes out to a little less than $200 per hour.

Administrator: That sounds about right. The room charge was $630, and the rest is pharmacy, supplies, laboratory, and ancillary services.

Me: That is quite a pharmacy bill! Is that what a pharmacy outside the hospital would charge for these services and supplies? I really think this bill must be padded.

Administrator: We have strict ethical guidelines and processes.

Me: You should also know that your nurses were not accustomed to caring for the needs of a person with quadriplegia, and therefore my wife provided most of my personal care during my stay at your hospital.

Administrator: Your needs are highly specialized. You know that your insurer has agreed to pay your bill, and you are only responsible for the copayment.

Me: That is quite a copayment for one day. Just because my insurer is stupid enough to pay this doesn't mean that I am as well. I just returned from a seven-day cruise on one of the top cruise lines, which cost me $2,200 for my entire family of four. My nineteen hours in your hospital and six hours in your emergency room cost about twice as much. And to be honest with you, I enjoyed the cruise more. For example, while your food was definitely good by hospital standards, you did not serve any caviar, smoked salmon, lobster, or baked Alaska. Given your prices, this menu would not have been unreasonable. I think I would be less upset if at least you had provided massages or liposuction or something.

Administrator: I understand.

Me: So what are you going to do about this? This bill is outrageous.

Administrator: I will have to get back to you.

Chapter 22. AUTONOMY, Inc.:
The Right to Live and Die

/Mitchell Batavia, Brother/

Drew's pioneering work in the right-to-die debate and physician-assisted dying controversy from a disability perspective was a hot-button topic and one that he saw as an extension of civil rights of persons with disabilities—the right for control over one's life, including a personal decision to end it.[1]

His perspective on this controversy first took shape during his painful recovery following his spinal cord injury, when he was anxious about whether he would have to endure unending pain and discomfort for the rest of his life. What gave him peace of mind, however, was the notion that if life became too unbearable, he could end it along with his suffering. Apparently, he discovered others in the disability community who thought along similar lines. Drew later solidified his position on physician-assisted dying when he contracted the flu, had difficulty breathing, and was rushed to an emergency room. What if the terror he felt while gasping for breath was not a short-term event, Drew reflected, but instead was part of an unending terminal condition? Under those circumstances, he would want the right to access a physician to help end his suffering, without government interference.[2]

Drew's perspective was also influenced by the loss of three friends with physical disabilities. Their lives became so unbearable that they decided to end them. They succeeded, unassisted, but with difficulty, sometimes requiring multiple tries due to botched earlier attempts. One of his friends with a poor quality of life, despite good resources, threw himself off the roof of his apartment building after two earlier self-inflicted attempts by stabbing (he could not grasp the knife adequately due to paralysis).[3] Another friend ended his life with a gun, and a third with an overdose of drugs.[4] Their final moments were likely not peaceful, and physician assistance could have been a great help.

In cases like these, Drew was ambivalent about whether persons with disabilities, those who are not terminally ill and not on life support, should be assisted in dying. On balance, he considered that those who suffer terribly (and in similar ways to the terminally ill) could, under "certain limited circumstances" and with "extremely stringent safeguards," have the right to physician-assisted dying, where the alternative might be repeated self-inflicted attempts to end their lives and continued suffering.[5] He viewed this as compassionate support for those who could not adjust to their disabilities, even when they were provided with alternative ways to live with dignity.[6]

On the other hand, Drew was far less ambivalent when it came to assisted dying for the terminally ill.[7] In the mid-1990s, he had the opportunity to advocate for mentally competent individuals who were terminally ill and sought medically assisted deaths. He did this pro bono work, which involved filing amicus briefs, while at his Florida law firm, McDermott Will & Emery. Drew authored and served as the attorney of record for a number of these briefs (where he was supportive but not directly connected to a particular case). His work included the US Supreme Court cases *Washington v. Glucksberg* and *Vacco v. Quill* in 1996 and the Florida Supreme Court case *Krischer v. McIver* in 1997.[8] These efforts were consistent with Drew's ongoing mission to safeguard the rights of people with disabilities, in this case, those who were terminally ill.

This work prompted Drew to launch AUTONOMY, Inc., a not-for-profit organization he cofounded to continue his mission of representing people with disabilities who wanted choices and control over their lives, including end-of-life decisions.[9] He established this organization in 2002, the year prior to his death.

Hugh Gallagher, vice president of AUTONOMY, defined its mission less delicately:

> AUTONOMY believes disabled people must take control of their own lives, free from the influence of doctors, social workers, nursing home directors, patronizing legislators, and all the other evildoers and do-gooders who have for so long bedeviled the lives of disabled people.

Drew assembled a board of directors, launched a website, and cultivated a strong following of more than 5,000. That year, the organization filed an amicus brief in the case of *Oregon v. Ashcroft*,[10] in support of the Death with Dignity Act, whereby terminally ill, mentally competent adults could achieve a peaceful death with the aid of physician-prescribed medication. In 2003, only the state of Oregon supported this right; since then, four additional states have joined the ranks: Vermont, Washington, California, and Montana (by court decision), and a county in New Mexico.[11] The rules vary among states, but in general, to meet the criteria, individuals must be terminally ill and have less than six months to live. Physicians cannot be prosecuted.

> *"Our society will have to address the views of people with disabilities, who have strong opinions on both sides of this issue."*

Drew's support of physician-assisted dying was likely the most contentious of his career, causing a rift in the disability community. Those against this right, such as a group called Not Dead Yet, used the slippery-slope argument that physicians who devalue persons with disabilities will opt to put them to death, given the chance. They referenced Nazi atrocities and suggested that states might find it cheaper to kill than to treat them, if the act became law.[12] One basis for their argument is that ending someone's life is wrong.[13]

On the other hand, Drew and others in AUTONOMY argued for persons with disabilities to make their own end-of-life decisions, free from state intrusion, and based on the principles of self-determination and autonomy. He argued that data from the Netherlands did not confirm Not Dead Yet's slippery-slope hypothesis, and that the Nazi analogy was off the mark, as these criminals instituted involuntary euthanasia. Indeed, Drew insisted that safeguards would be in place and that individuals who wanted them would not be giving up any of their protective rights to stay alive.[14] For a comprehensive account of both groups' arguments, see Quill and Battin's *Physician-Assisted Dying: The Case for*

Palliative Care and Patient Choice[15] and Foley and Hendin's *The Case Against Assisted Suicide: For the Right to End-of-Life Care.*[16]

These two groups—each unpacking arguments to support disability rights—just opposed each other.[17] Members of Not Dead Yet even demonstrated outside the US Supreme Court while Drew presented an amicus brief in favor of the right to assisted dying.[18] Although I wasn't present during these court confrontations, I could only imagine Drew standing tall on his principles while a segment of the disability community wanted him sitting down.

Cheryl recalls the group referring to Drew as "elite," someone who had the advantages of a wonderful education, financial resources, and enough influence to prevent some doctor from deciding that his quality of life was so poor that he should die. She also told me Drew was distressed about the hard feelings within the disability-rights community surrounding this issue and was working on an article to heal the rift around the time of his death.

While the disability community is divided over physician-assisted dying, Drew highlighted areas of agreement. First, most people in the disability community agree they have experienced a long history of devaluation by society, accompanied by discrimination and prejudices. Second, our health care system, with its cost-cutting measures, has disproportionately impacted the disability community, who may rely on services most. Some fear this may encourage a practice of helping people die; others believe a universal health care system can address this issue. Finally, both sides agree that there is the potential for abuses in physician-assisted dying. While some believe effective safeguards address this concern, others do not.[19]

Drew believed the controversy of physician-assisted dying would not simply disappear. He wrote, "Our society will have to address the views of people with disabilities, who have strong opinions on both sides of this issue."[20]

Chapter 23. The Final Two Years

/Mitchell Batavia, Brother/

During the last two years of Drew's life, he became sick more often and more severely. This was despite ramped-up productivity at work and dedicated parenting at home. He was really just holding on for the kids. Although he scrupulously attended to his health, he was losing the fight.

He even told Joe one day, "I'm trying very hard to live. I want to be here for you."

Even eighteen months before his death, while Drew traveled to New York City with his family for my wedding at the Russian Tea Room, he was not well. We took him to Rusk to have him evaluated by a physiatrist and a urologist because he was uncomfortable and complained of persistent muscle spasms that he couldn't shake, another urinary tract infection.

And then there was his July 2002 hospitalization for a urinary tract infection just prior to taking a cruise with his family, about six months before he died, and another hospitalization at Mount Sinai Medical Center in Florida in December, about a week before his death. He may have been fighting pneumonia as well.

I was not aware of how seriously his health had deteriorated during those last months, though, like many of us, I was in denial. I had viewed a documentary about his family, filmed about three months before his death. I watched it with my mom at her home in Boynton Beach, along with Cheryl and the kids shortly after his death, and then again at Drew's memorial service. I was stunned to see the degree of weight loss and the effort he made to steal air so that he could complete a full sentence during his interview. A superbug had established residency.

Drew may have sensed it too, perhaps during conversations with his physicians, as he frequented them more often. His wife tells me, "He worked feverishly on his memoirs late into the night, as if racing time." And in those latter years, even when we visited or talked on the phone, the subject of health came up.

I even recall that, during one visit, we were sitting in a café on Lincoln Road, a promenade of posh shops, art galleries, and people watching in South Beach. We were having a casual chat, plotting out future projects—he was always planning new projects. Then he stared at me, and said with a straight face, "You know, I don't want to live forever." I thought the comment strange and out of character for someone with his fervent ambition and vision. In retrospect, I should have asked him to elaborate, but at the time, I didn't give it serious consideration. He took care of himself. He took precautions. He always bounced back. Denial.

While reflecting on Drew's achievements, and mostly during the writing of this memoir, I arrived at an epiphany. Drew's life seemed to mirror the fictional armored character, Don Quixote of La Mancha, a fighter for justice. Was this just a coincidence? Was the seventeenth-century Spanish novel written by Miguel de Cervantes Saavedra more than just a passing literary inspiration for Drew? Did it serve as a model for living? Drew battled for the civil rights of a group of people who, for the most part, were not well represented.

And yet during his life, I was shamefully clueless about who the postaccident Drew really was. Even at family gatherings, he would pepper conversations with applying for a White House Fellowship, writing an amicus brief, or launching a website called Autonomy-now.org. But it was just over most of our heads. My knee-jerk response at holiday dinners went something like, "That's wonderful, Drew, would you like some more turkey?" How obtuse was I!

To be fair, Drew did not broadcast accomplishments. In fact, when he moved back to Yonkers in 1974, he shared with me a disturbing incident in which someone breached his confidence, sharing information he preferred to remain private. While talking in his bedroom, he offered me advice: "Be very careful who you share with." He said this with a lasting, wounded stare. True to form, he did not share the details of this breach with me either. I never forgot this cryptic conversation and now wonder if Drew may have developed a general tendency, since that time, of holding back information he did not feel comfortable releasing. Or perhaps he would be discreet with whom he did share. In any case, we may have been working with missing information during Drew's ladder climb.

We would hear pieces and bits about his job and read his celebrated holiday letters, but the many pieces of his life never came together, at least for me. He was family, my big brother, my bunk buddy, not a government gadfly. Like the viewer of an optical illusion, I could see only the image I was familiar with, the polite wallflower, not the alternative one, a policy pugilist.

But that was my problem, not his. *I never let go of the past; he did.* My yearning to trade places with him, at any cost, to appease his hell and perhaps my self-inflicted guilt, so Drew could be Drew again, is evidence that I never really accepted his injury. Yet he did. How's that for irony?

Drew adjusted famously to his life in a wheelchair. In fact, many with quadriplegia do so within about a year of their injury, but Drew was exceptional. I'll never forget how we watched news coverage of Christopher Reeve, famed for his role as Superman and also for breaking his neck in a freak riding accident, logging hundreds of hours of exercise, using therapeutic pools and treadmills, and hiring what seemed like an army of physical therapists, in an attempt to walk again. It never happened. After the news coverage, Drew, with the timing of Groucho Marx, turned to me and said, "I don't believe I was ever that delusional." Even so, the depth of Drew's commitment to his newly adopted lifestyle is something I never quite got, a life that he continued to say he would never trade with anyone.

And yet, despite having high-level quadriplegia, Drew never viewed himself as a person with a disability. My mom even relayed a curious story of when she and my dad were visiting Drew while he was an undergraduate at the University of California, Riverside.

> We were out to dinner and were approached by a waiter who called Drew by name. Seeing the quizzical look on Drew's face, the waiter said, "Don't you remember me? I was a teacher assistant in your econ class last semester." Drew, of course, acknowledged him, and they chatted for a few minutes. When he left, Drew said, "I really can't place him. I wonder how come he recognized me?"

I did notice a fundamental change in Drew following his injury, and it wasn't just physical. Whenever Drew was in the room with us, I sensed he was also somewhere else, mildly distracted, tolerantly aloof, quietly prioritizing. His attention seemed split. It's as if he had a vision, orchestrating some mission, but was not quite ready to share it with the rest of us. Drew was plotting.

All this led me to an incontrovertible, and surprisingly obvious, conclusion: Drew was the Don Quixote in the wheelchair.

As I see it, Drew left the nondisabled world years ago, at the time of the car wreck, and he never looked back. In a sense, he died that night in 1973 and resurfaced within a community that needed him desperately, laid claim to him, and that he now belonged to, the disability community. And for this community, he found life purpose. He saw how individuals with disabilities were not given the same opportunities and rights as others. He became a guardian, a fighter for equal rights for health care and at work, for building access and during travel, while living and when dying. He fought for ramps and curb cuts, insurance coverage and work accommodations, and perhaps the most important decision in one's life: how to end it.

Certainly, his work benefited his community. But who doesn't know someone with a disability? Eventually each one of us will likely inherit, if not "procure," a malady that will impede our function as we age. In fact, the disability community is the largest minority in America. And it favors not one religion, race, ethnicity, or political group over any other. It matters little whether you are a Kennedy or a Reagan, black or white, a Catholic or a Jew. And Drew fought for all of them—the forlorn, the uninformed, and the not-yet-born—so that all these individuals can experience as full a life as those without disabilities.

All this led me to an incontrovertible, and surprisingly obvious, conclusion:

Drew was the Don Quixote in the wheelchair. He came to this role in the same way his teenage brilliance arrived: modestly.

But this is not just a story about Drew and his mission. His memoirs hold a universal message about our human capacity to achieve things worthwhile. With insatiable drive and unfettered vision, many of us are capable of the extraordinary. This may even be truer for those who have a disability and are forced to pull from their residual resources, as was the case with Drew. Other examples include the political acumen of Franklin Delano Roosevelt, who had paraplegia; the brilliant physics of Stephen Hawking, who has ALS; and, more recently, the baffling feat of Jean-Dominique Bauby, the editor in chief of *Elle* who dictated his memoir, *The Diving Bell and the Butterfly*, following a severe stroke, solely by blinking one eye. In all these cases, whatever remained in these individuals was maximally directed toward astonishing productivity. Can we learn from them? Is it possible to fully exploit what we already possess within ourselves? Conceivably, each one of us can emerge as a Don Quixote.

Near the time I was planning to help complete Drew's memoirs, Cheryl shared a striking conversation she had with Drew. Shortly before he died, Drew said to Cheryl, "Nobody appreciates me."

"Everybody appreciates you, Drew," she replied. "I appreciate you."

"Yes, you probably do appreciate me more than most people do," he said, "but most people only know me in one area of my life."

I think what Drew was getting at was that no one person fully grasped the totality of his accomplishments—and I think he was right. Even top scholars familiar with one area of Drew's work were clueless of other neighboring pursuits Drew was deeply engaged in.

> *"No person, living or dead, has done more for the civil rights of people with disabilities than had Drew."*

He was in the forefront of ADA regulations, the right-to-die debate, the independent living and the personal assistant national service movements. He was involved in politics and law, an expert in health care research and finance, and engaged in journal article publication, university teaching, national committee work, and nonprofit organizations. And he was an entrepreneur, a book author, a newspaper column writer, a poet, a husband, and a papa.

I can't remember the exact quote about legacies, but it goes something like this: A measure of your life corresponds to the number of people you touch. Drew touched legions of people through his activism, professing, theorizing, writing, regulating, litigating, befriending, and parenting. And through his efforts he helped the underserved. This is not to say there were no other movers and shakers within the disability community; there were, in great numbers. Some were his friends, like Hugh Gallagher, an international disability advocate and historian. But Drew was in a particularly leveraged position, given his public and private appointments, his legal and policy training, his tenacity and impatience, his timing. As Hugh Gallagher wrote in a letter for Drew's memorial: "No person, living or dead, has done more for the civil rights of people with disabilities than had Drew."

Drew had a multifaceted, full life. You had to dive deep and wide to appreciate its ridiculously expansive reach. I spent a half-year pouring over his work to better grasp it. It was hard to keep up, and you had to be smart to do so. But this memoir is a remedy. It has been for me, and I hope it will be for you.

It is only fitting that Drew has the last word in his memoirs, quoted from his preface:

My mission in this world is to try to ensure that all people, including people with disabilities, have greater choices in and control over their lives. I believe that achieving this mission will make the world a slightly better place than it was before I got here.

Chapter 24. Postscript: The Memorial Service

/Mitchell Batavia, Brother/

On January 6, 2003, Drew passed away peacefully, with dignity, and in the manner he wished, at Jackson Memorial Hospital in Florida. His life was celebrated at a memorial service a week later at Beth Israel Memorial Chapel in Delray Beach. The service was attended by more than 200 people. Pews overflowed and unseated guests stood near the rear, peering through a gaping propped-open door. Letters flew in from all corners of the US and as far away as the Netherlands, from friends, colleagues, dignitaries. I briefly summarized Drew's life accomplishments at the opening of the service; my father, Gabriel, led the assemblage in a prayer, the Kaddish, at the closing. And in between, guests shared true tales of an incredible and big life. They shared Drew stories.

The Order of Speakers:
Mitchell Batavia (brother)
Renée Batavia (mother)
Cheryl Batavia (wife)
Joe Batavia (son)
Katey Batavia (daughter)
Mitchell Batavia (brother)

Gabriel Batavia (father)

Marian Nicholson (mother-in-law)

Ellen Maher (Cheryl's daughter): Letters from Curt Nicholson (Cheryl's brother) and Melody Jorgenson (Cheryl's niece)

Beverly Silverman (aunt)

Dean Berkman (dean, FIU)

Gerben DeJong (colleague, director NRH Research Center)

Jennifer Fabré and Rob Simone (U Miami students; documentary of Drew and his family)

Donna Batavia (sister): Letter from Dick and Ginny Thornburgh, former attorney general of the United States and his wife

Sheri and Paul Pierson (cousins)

Mitchell Batavia (brother): Letter from Vice Admiral John W. Miller (1990-1991 White House Fellow) and Mary Pat Miller

Rhonda Kessler (cousin)

Gerben DeJong: Letter from Victor Fuchs, Stanford professor emeritus

David Brush (cousin)

Thomas James Maher (husband of Ellen Maher): Letter from Senator John McCain

Donna Batavia (sister): Letter from Senator Sam Brownback (1990-1991 White House Fellow)

David Brush (cousin): Letter from Hugh Gallagher

Sonia Mitchell (principal of Florida International Academy, where Cheryl taught)

Cheryl Batavia (wife): Letter from James Cadigan (Drew's personal assistant)

Louise Bauer (cousin)

Gerben DeJong (colleague): Letter from Anthony Principi, secretary of Veterans Affairs; letter from Edward A. Eckenhoff , president and CEO of National Rehabilitation Hospital
Mary Margolius (cousin)
Cheryl Batavia (wife): Letter from Jody Greenstone Miller (1990-1991 White House Fellow)
Bob Grusky: Letter from Rob Chess (both are 1990-1991 White House Fellows)
Gabriel Batavia (father): Kaddish

Included below are speeches by Drew's children, who spoke at the service:

Friends and family, we're here today to say goodbye to Papa. Papa helped a lot of people. If Dad hadn't had his accident, he would never have met Mama, and they never would have adopted us. Papa was a good friend to everyone. He worked very late on his computer writing books, and he still had lots of time to spend with his family and friends. He helped Katey and me learn to read. He always stuck around when we needed help. Papa always kept his promises. And never broke any promises. Papa wanted me to be responsible and be the man of the family, and I'm going to keep my promise. (Joe Batavia, age 12)

I love my daddy so much, like a rock. I always wear the blue polar bear shirt he likes. I always ask him if he would come outside and play with me. He says later, and then he plays with me. I give him lots of hugs, and sometimes I help him do his grades. He helped me with my homework, and he always calls me a "monkey face." I read a lot of books to him. On Saturday and Sunday we watch Channel 6 together, and I help Papa get up. I like to go to the park and Lincoln Road with my daddy. I get my dad's tea, and I give it to him. I always do the boxes on my dad's computer, because he needs help with that. I miss my daddy, and I want to grow up like my daddy. (Katey Batavia, age 10)

Endnotes

Preface
1. At the time of his writing, Drew planned on writing a second volume.

Chapter 1
1. This name is a pseudonym.

Chapter 4
1. To protect confidentiality, the names of the patients in this chapter have been changed.
2. The names Cupid and Alfred in this section are pseudonyms.
3. Without reviewing Drew's original medical record, I could not verify whether his stated level of injury was vertebral or neurologic.
4. Maxim J. McKibben, Patrick Seed, Sherry S. Ross, and Kristy M. Borawski, "Urinary Tract Infection and Neurogenic Bladder," *Urologic Clinics of North America* 42, no. 4 (2015): 527-36.
5. Andrew I. Batavia, "Of Wheelchairs and Managed Care," *Health Affairs* 18, no. 6 (1999): 177-82.

Chapter 9
1. Drew's writing predated Eliot Spitzer's election as governor of New York and subsequent resignation.
2. After Drew's death, Tim Kaine became governor of Virginia, chairman of the Democratic National Committee, and a US Senator.

Chapter 11
1. The names Michael and Alan in this section are pseudonyms.

Chapter 12
1. Dr. Toerge was medical director at the time Drew wrote his memoirs.
2. Andrew I. Batavia, "Representation and Role Separation in the Disability Movement: Should Researchers Be Advocates?" *Archives of Physical Medicine and Rehabilitation* 70, no. 4 (1989): 345-48.

Chapter 13
1. Colin Powell was secretary of state at the time of Drew's writing.

Chapter 14
1. ADA regulations, Title III, Part 36, Nondiscrimination on the basis of disability by public accommodations and in commercial facilities, http://www.ada.gov/reg3a.html#anchor-36000
2. "A Celebration of the 25th Anniversary of the Americans with Disabilities Act," http://www.ada.gov/ada_25th_anniversary/25th_event_livevi deo.html

3. Dick Thornburgh, "The Disabilities Revolution," *Pittsburgh Post-Gazette,* May 3, 2015, http://www.post-gazette.com/opinion/Op-Ed/2015/05/03/Dick-Thornburgh-The-revolution-created-by-the-Americans-with-Disabilities-Act/stories/201505030151

Chapter 15
1. "George H. W. Bush Calls Americans with Disabilities Act One of His Proudest Achievements," https://www.looktothestars.org/news/13990-george-h-w-bush-calls-americans-with-disabilities-act-one-of-his-proudest-achievements

Chapter 18
1. Sofia Khan, Mary Plummer, Alberto Martinez-Arizala, and Kresimir Banovac, "Hypothermia in Patients with Chronic Spinal Cord Injury," *The Journal of Spinal Cord Medicine* 30, no. 1 (2007): 27-30.

Chapter 21
1. A. I. Batavia, "A disability rights-independent living perspective on euthanasia," *Western Journal of Medicine* 154, no. 5 (May 1991): 616-617.
2. Andrew I. Batavia, *Independent Living: A Viable Option for Long-Term Care* (Clearwater, Florida: ABI Professional Publications, 2003).
3. Andrew I. Batavia, "Accounting for the Health-Care Bill," *The Lancet* 362, no. 9394 (2003): 1495-97.

Chapter 22
1. A. I. Batavia, "A disability rights-independent living perspective on euthanasia," *Western Journal of Medicine* 154, no. 5 (May 1991): 616-617.

2. Andrew Batavia, comments in conference transcript, "Socially Assisted Dying: Media, Money, and Meaning," *Cornell Journal of Law and Public Policy* 7, no. 2 (Winter 1998): 274-78, 292-93, 348-49, 394-96.

3. Ibid.

4. Andrew I. Batavia, "The Relevance of Data on Physicians and Disability on the Right to Assisted Suicide: Can Empirical Studies Resolve the Issue?" *Psychology, Public Policy, and Law* 6, no. 2 (June 2000), 546-558.

5. Ibid.

6. Andrew I. Batavia, "Disability and Physician-Assisted Dying" in *Physician-Assisted Dying: The Case for Palliative Care and Patient Choice*, edited by Timothy E. Quill and Margaret P. Battin (Baltimore: Johns Hopkins University Press, 2004), 55-74.

7. Alternative terms used in this debate include "physician-assisted suicide," "physician aid in dying," "aid in dying," "assisted dying," and "death with dignity."

8. See Appendix G ("Pro Bono Appellate & Supreme Court Experience").

9. Batavia, "Disability and Physician-Assisted Dying."

10. See Appendix G.

11. "Physician-Assisted Suicide Fast Facts," October 6, 2015, http://www.cnn.com/2014/11/26/us/physician-assisted-suicide-fast-facts/

12. Batavia, "Disability and Physician-Assisted Suicide."

13. Quill and Battin, *Physician-Assisted Dying*.

14. Batavia, "Disability and Physician-Assisted Suicide."

15. Quill and Battin, *Physician-Assisted Dying*.

16. Kathleen M. Foley and Herbert Hendin, eds., *The Case Against Assisted Suicide: For the Right to End-of-Life Care* (Baltimore: Johns Hopkins University Press, 2002).

17. Batavia, "Disability and Physician-Assisted Suicide."

18. Rosenberg, Carol. "Miamian Fights for the Ill's Right to Choose Death," *Miami Herald,* page 9A, January 9, 1997.
19. Batavia, "Disability and Physician-Assisted Suicide."
20. Ibid.

Appendix E
1. I should clarify this statement at the outset, lest I lose part of my readership at this very early stage of this book. There are two aspects of political correctness, one of which is positive and the other of which is very negative. The positive aspect relates to a sensitivity to diversity and a commitment to characterize people with different racial and other characteristics as they would like to be characterized and to treat them with the respect that all people should be treated. The negative aspect of political correctness concerns an obligation to conform to certain accepted "truths" because they are regarded as politically desirable, whether or not they are empirically accurate. I believe that we should pursue the truth irrespective of where it takes us, and that we must communicate truths in a respectful, but entirely intellectually honest, manner.

Appendix G
1. Drew was also a speaker at conferences of the Centers for Disease Control, the National Head Injury Foundation, and several other national groups addressing issues of health care reform.

Appendix A.
Timeline

June 1957   Born in Brooklyn

1966   Moved to Yonkers

1973   Yonkers Marathon
Summer Counselor
Accident
Montefiore Acute Hospital, Bronx

1974   Rehabilitation at Rusk, New York City

1975   Return to Yonkers
Graduated Lincoln High School

1975-1976   University of California, Berkeley

1976-1980   BA, University of California, Riverside

1980-1982   Harvard Law School

1982   1982 Summer associate, Fried, Frank,
Harris, Shriver & Jacobson

1980-1983	MS in health services research, Stanford University Medical School
1983-1984	Stanford Law School
1984	JD, Harvard Law School
1984-1986	Attorney, US Department of Health and Human Services
1984	Hired Cheryl
1986-1987	Mary E. Switzer Distinguished Research Fellowship
1987-1989	Assoc. director, health services research, National Rehabilitation Hospital
1990-1991	White House Fellowship Special assistant to the attorney general, US Department of Justice
1991	Marriage to Cheryl
1991-1992	Senior staff, White House Domestic Policy Council
1992-1993	Research director for disability and rehab policy, ABT Associates
1993	Executive director, National Council on Disability

1993-1995	Legislative assistant, Office of US Senator John McCain
1995	Speaker, UC Riverside Commencement
1995-1997	Counsel, McDermott Will & Emery
1996	Adoption of Joe and Katey
1997	Associate professor, Florida International University Founder, AUTONOMY, Inc.
July 2002	Last cruise
January 6, 2003	Death
January 2003	Tenure and promotion to full professor (posthumous)

Appendix B.
Lessons Learned

Drew cultivated a life philosophy while in a wheelchair, one he wished to share in these memoirs. Many of these lessons are hinted at below in his table of contents for Part 2, which he never got around to writing. Nevertheless, he would have likely highlighted the following tenets, which can be culled from the completed portion (Part 1). Included are: the importance of an enduring vision, a high sense of purpose, an indefatigable ethic of long work days, a strong moral compass, impatience, honesty (he was not particularly interested in being politically correct), a self-deprecating sense of humor, life checklists, and an attitude of not taking anything for granted, not even a single day. Drew took jobs to learn and then moved on to learn more. He took calculated risks, pushing himself to his physical limits (for example, sitting and typing for ten to fourteen hours) before risking the development of a pressure ulcer. He weighed opportunities, possibly using a decision-making process similar to Benjamin Franklin's, listing pros and cons. Importantly, the Don Quixote mission of righting wrongs and Friedrich Nietzsche's aphorism, "What does not kill me makes me stronger," served Drew well during his life.

Table of Contents for Part 2 of the Memoir (Unfinished)

Appendix C.
UC Riverside Commencement Address, 1995

Andrew I. Batavia, JD, MS

Chancellor Orbach, Vice Chancellor Erickson, faculty members, graduates, families, and friends, this occasion brings back very fond memories for me. It was just fifteen years ago, in June 1980, that I was on this platform receiving my bachelor's degree. That day marked the successful conclusion of perhaps the most challenging period of my life, and the beginning of a new set of challenges that would not have been possible if not for the preparation I received at UC Riverside.

Just seven years earlier, in August 1973, I broke my neck in an auto accident in which I was thrown through the windshield from the backseat of the car. This is a feat that I would not recommend to anyone. I spent the following year in a sequence of intensive care, acute care, and rehabilitation facilities. I completed my junior year of high school while in rehabilitation, thereby allowing me to graduate in 1975 with the same class with which I shared my freshman and sophomore years.

That year, the major topic of conversation among seniors at Lincoln High School in Yonkers, New York, like at other high schools throughout the nation, was which colleges we would be applying to. For me, this turned out to be a relatively easy decision. I was informed early in the process that there were only four schools in the entire country that could accommodate the needs associated with my disability: the University of Illinois; the University of Miami; UC Berkeley; and UC Riverside.

Illinois seemed to me uninhabitable for at least eight months of the year. Miami offered too many distractions for the stoic intellectual pursuit of knowledge. Everyone had heard of Berkeley, and no one had heard of Riverside. While I was told that UC Riverside was a great place to go to school, I decided instead to go with the greater prestige of Berkeley. This proved to be an unfortunate decision!

My first official action at Berkeley was to roll off a sidewalk in an unsuccessful attempt to climb one of the campus's many hills that were too steep for my wheelchair. In retrospect, I should have regarded this as an omen.

The various trials and tribulations I underwent during my freshman year are too many to relate here, but may be summarized in aggregate as a "character-building experience" for a young person who was 3,000 miles from home, who had never before lived independently, and who was just learning to cope with his disability. There just were not the strong support structures at a big school like Berkeley that would have helped that transition. I relate this not to criticize Berkeley, which is a great school, but to point out the even greater strengths of UCR.

The low point of my freshman year at Berkeley was the last day of my Anthropology 1 course. The professor, who usually departed through the back door at the end of class, decided to make a dramatic exit up the long flight of lecture hall stairs. Situated at the top step, where my wheelchair was parked throughout the course, this gave me my first opportunity to see this professor up close and exchange a few words with him. I waited patiently as he slowly ascended the stairs. Finally, as he approached the top step, I told him how much I enjoyed the course. To which he nodded "Thanks" and disappeared.

The next day I found myself calling UC Riverside for a transfer application. I just decided that I wanted a more personalized undergraduate education. When I made that life-changing phone call, I had to repeat my request several times to the administrator on the phone line. Apparently, at the time, UCR did not receive many requests for transfers *from* Berkeley. The following September, I was on this beautiful campus. It turned out to be one of the best decisions I ever made.

At UCR, I received the personal attention I needed to grow. The classes were small, at least by Berkeley standards, and I knew many of my professors. I often think about this intimate, caring academic environment which fostered both my intellectual and personal development. Among my best memories are of attending debates between the radical and conservative economists competing for our "young, impressionable" minds, going to the Barn to listen to great performers like Elizabeth Cotton, and partying with friends at the Aberdeen-Inverness dorms. While the campus has grown substantially since I was a student. I am pleased to find that UCR maintains its warm and friendly charm.

Since I left UCR in 1980, its lessons have continued to serve me well. The school prepared me for rigorous academic programs at Harvard Law School, Stanford Medical School, and Stanford Law School. It taught me to think critically and independently, and to question conventional wisdom. While this capacity occasionally gets me in trouble, it generally has been appreciated by my colleagues. Overall, my UCR education enhanced my ability to formulate and organize my thoughts and to communicate them to a wider audience. These skills have since helped me greatly in both my government and private-sector work.

It is traditional for a commencement speaker to offer some wise insights to provide direction for the future. Because this is my first time doing this, it seems premature to break tradition. So, I would like to focus my insights on the theme of growth, a topic which seems appropriate as we celebrate the passage of our graduates to the next stage of their lives, having grown along with UCR over the past few years. Both individuals and the institutions they create must be fostered to grow to fulfill their potentials.

To Chancellor Orbach and the administration, I applaud your many successes in expanding the scope and depth of this campus. It is of a much grander scale than when I attended, yet in many ways the same. Like your predecessors, you are fulfilling the great promise of UCR that was entrusted to you, and for that you have our gratitude. Let UCR continue to grow, as it must, in a manner that maintains its greatest attribute, its nurturing academic environment. We must never compromise that great strength.

To the faculty, including those professors who taught me when I was here, continue to offer the personal attention that you generously gave me and my fellow students. It may not seem so on a daily basis, but the long-term effects of such concern on the growth of your students are profound. I know this empirically through a fifteen-year longitudinal study I personally conducted of an admittedly small sample of UCR graduates, which, if not statistically significant, is profoundly relevant to our lives.

To families and friends, give your graduates the continued support and encouragement to pursue their dreams. In the ten years since I graduated law school, I have achieved the dubious distinction of having pursued five different careers— as an attorney, a health services researcher, a consultant, a public administrator, and a legislative assistant. I also hold the unofficial UCR record for the most changes of majors as an undergraduate, having refiled on the average of every other week during my sophomore year. While my parents often joke with me about this, and frequently ask when I am going to get a real job, they never discouraged me. For this, I will always be grateful.

And finally, to the graduates, set your goals high and strive to surpass them. Dream big and dare to succeed! You will achieve beyond your expectations. It is easy to be overwhelmed by the enormity of the working world in which you are about to enter (or to postpone through graduate studies). It is too easy to conclude that the great institutions of our society have little need for someone who is recently out of school, who has little or no real-world experience, and who will require their time and resources to train.

The fact is these organizations desperately need good people and the competent and ethical leadership they provide. They particularly need people like you with the ability to apply theory and knowledge to the practical problems that confront them. They need people like you with the mental agility to learn to function quickly and effectively, and the confidence in themselves to take calculated risks. The bottom line is that, as much as you need them, they need you to survive and flourish in an increasingly complex and competitive global environment.

Once you have found your organization, seek out mentors and role models to help you learn the ropes and avoid the pitfalls. I have benefitted from several remarkable people who have invested in my development. With the help of such individuals, figure out how the organization can be improved. Then, work to make the necessary changes. If you are so inclined, establish your own organizations to do the job better. Your only limitations are those which you impose on yourselves. I know from personal experience that all perceived obstacles can be surmounted.

Most important, maintain perspective! I never cease to be amazed over the number of high achievers at institutions where I have studied and worked, including Harvard, Stanford, the Justice Department, and the White House, who have lost track of who they are and what they have achieved. In fact, I have on occasion been guilty of this myself. Know your goals and your priorities. Decide what you want to achieve during your lifetime; how and for what you want to be remembered. Recognize that while productive time is necessary, so is leisure time: time with the people who are important to you.

Always remember the person you are and the person you ultimately want to grow to be. And surround yourself with good friends and family members who will remind you when you forget.

You are the beneficiaries of the finest education that our nation offers, and you will provide the expertise and leadership our country needs. Find happiness and fulfillment. We are all very proud of you. Congratulations, and thank you for this wonderful opportunity to return to UCR.

Appendix D.
White House Fellowship Application Essay

MEMORANDUM

Date: December 3, 1989

To: The President

From: Andrew Batavia

Re: **A National Attendant Services Program for Americans with Disabilities**

<u>Background</u>

Through our successes in medicine, we have created a growing challenge to our social insurance and health care systems. There are approximately two million Americans with physical disabilities severe enough to require paid attendant services. Although their disabilities vary, a common denominator among many of these persons is that they:
- need assistance to conduct their daily activities;
- prefer to obtain such assistance while living in their homes, not in institutions;

- cannot afford to pay for such assistance with their own resources; and
- cannot locate dependable assistants even if they could afford them.

The Problem

There are three likely negative consequences for disabled persons whose needs are not met:

- The individual will be unable to obtain gainful employment to assist the individual; and
- The individual will develop health problems, often resulting in expensive institutional care or death.

Most agree that, when feasible, it is preferable to provide assistance to disabled persons in the community rather than in institutions. Further, home-based assistance is likely to generate large savings for society. Yet, the US has no policy on home-based assistance for disabled persons. To the extent there is any national disability policy on long-term care, it focuses on financing expensive medical services provided through home health agencies and nursing homes.

Proposed Solutions

The primary legislative approach to developing a national attendant services program has been to expand the Medicare and Medicaid programs. A few bills such as the "Medicare Long-Term Home Care Catastrophic Protection Act of 1988" and the "Lifecare Long-Term Protection Act of 1988" have provided for coverage of home-based attendant services. While these bills have merit, they tend to be expensive ($8-40 billion per year) and do not address the problem of recruitment of attendants.

An alternative approach is to finance and recruit attendants as part of a National Service Corps program. Among the bills to develop such a program are the "Citizenship and National Service Act of 1989." In return for full-time community service, high school graduates would receive a living stipend and a voucher for college, vocational training, or a first home.

This approach would address the need for attendant services while providing job experience and economic opportunity. Relying on recent high school graduates, it is likely to be less expensive than the health care bills cited above and would directly address the problem of recruitment. Moreover, this approach strongly supports the "thousand points of light" theme of your presidential campaign. With your leadership, it is likely to receive bipartisan support.

Recommendation

I recommend that a National Service Corps approach to meeting the assistance needs of disabled persons be seriously considered, and that we either support one of the existing bills before Congress or develop an alternative bill.

Appendix E.
Resurrecting the Bull Moose

(originally Part 1, Chapter 23)

Drew's views on politics evolved. Resurrecting the Bull Moose Party reflects a change in Drew's political orientation during the last two years of his life, a philosophy more in line with one of his heroes, Theodore Roosevelt, who founded it. Roosevelt had become weary with America's two-party system and wanted to resurrect a party that stood for honesty. From his writings, Drew planned to write a book on this topic. What follows is the preface to that work.

The Party's Over:
Ending the Democrat-Republican Conspiracy
Against the American Public

Andrew I. Batavia, JD, MS

Preface
"I am a Bull Moose." That is my reply nowadays when asked to identify my political party, alluding to the reform party under which Theodore Roosevelt pursued a third term

for president in 1912. Like millions of other Americans, I have given up all hope of our two-party system in providing the leadership our country needs. Unlike most other Americans, I have had the privilege of observing this system at a fairly high level, and therefore am well positioned to assess its various strengths and weaknesses. This book is about those strengths and weaknesses, why the American public is poorly served by the Democratic and Republican parties, and how we can and must fix our flawed political system.

One's political affiliation, to the extent that one is willing to affiliate with a political party, depends upon a variety of cultural, socioeconomic, and other considerations. I believe one key factor is when the individual gained political consciousness—the time in life when people begin to perceive themselves as political beings who are part of a broader political context. For example, those who achieved political consciousness during FDR's New Deal have a substantial likelihood of identifying themselves as lifelong Democrats. Those achieving political consciousness during the Reagan administration are more likely to be strong Republicans. Although this theory must be tested empirically, it appears to have some validity based upon anecdotal experience.

I became politically conscious fairly late in life—at about twenty years of age— at least compared with many of my peers who had older siblings or who came from more politically involved families. Many of them achieved political consciousness in their teenage years during the Nixon administration, with the Vietnam War and the Watergate scandal. Raised in a liberal suburb of New York City, almost all became lifelong Democrats at a very young age. Although I am slightly embarrassed now over having matured politically so late, I believe this has been beneficial to me, in that it did not ossify my political thought processes at an early age. My thoughts were not restricted by notions of "political correctness" that limit the thinking of many of my contemporaries.[1]

I achieved political consciousness during the Carter administration. This was the time in our nation's history in which we were experiencing stagflation—extremely high inflation and interest rates in conjunction with very high unemployment rates associated with an economic recession—while we were waiting on long lines to gas stations and watching Americans held hostage in Iran for over a year. Coming to political consciousness at this particular point in time guaranteed that I could never be a Democrat for the remainder of my life, despite the fact that I come from a long line of lifetime Democrats.

My disaffection with the Republican Party took a much longer period of time to develop and a much more circuitous route. I was actually registered as an independent until the age of thirty-three. I never particularly liked how we treat politics in this country like a football game, in which there are two teams intent upon winning at virtually any cost, even if our nation does not necessarily share in the victory. Moreover, professionally, as a researcher who addressed health care, disability, and other social issues affected by the political system, I thought it preferable to avoid party affiliation rather than having my objectivity and credibility challenged on partisan political grounds. In 1990, however, an important development in my career induced me to choose sides.

That was the year I was selected as a White House Fellow. The White House Fellowship Program is a highly competitive program in which individuals among the top young prospects in their respective fields, including business, the military, and academia, are brought to Washington to serve and learn at the highest levels of the federal government. Specifically, each fellow is selected to serve as a special assistant to a cabinet member or high-ranking White House official. Among the fellows who have since risen to national acclaim are Secretary of State General Colin Powell, and US Senator Sam Brownback (who was a member of my fellowship class and a close friend despite our political differences).

After being selected as a fellow, I was recruited strongly by Attorney General of the United States Richard Thornburgh to be his special assistant. To this day, I do not know why he wanted me on board at the Justice Department, but I will always be grateful that he did. When I accepted his offer, I had an important decision to make; I could remain politically independent or become a Republican. The White House Fellows program is entirely nonpartisan, and every fellowship class has both Democrats and Republicans who serve the president and administration irrespective of political affiliation. Although I received no pressure whatsoever from Thornburgh or anyone else in the Bush administration (in fact, they do not even know about my independent affiliation), I decided to become a Republican at that time.

I chose to become a Republican for several reasons. First, as stated earlier, I could never be a Democrat after gaining political consciousness during the Carter administration. Second, I was attracted to several of the major principles of the Republican Party, particularly the commitment to fiscal responsibility and individual accountability. (That was back in the good old days, when Republicans actually stood for a balanced budget, and not just tax cuts, and the Republican

Party was the party of Main Street, and not just Wall Street.) Although I was and continue to be concerned about the influence of fundamentalist religious/social conservatives within the Republican Party, they did not seem to control the party at the time, and I recognized that in a two-party system one must learn to live with some strange bedfellows.

The third reason I decided to become a Republican was of a more personal nature. I developed an immediate admiration for Attorney General Thornburgh, who had already had a distinguished career as a federal prosecutor, prosecuting white-collar crime, and who, as the two-time governor of Pennsylvania, had managed the Three Mile Island nuclear plant crisis. I also had admiration for President Bush, who had worked his way up in the Republican Party to be President Reagan's successor and who had earned the presidency. With leaders such as these, and particularly Senator Bob Dole, I felt comfortable becoming a Republican at the time.

I remained a loyal and committed Republican for the next eleven years. Following my fellowship, I served on a detail to the staff of the White House Domestic Policy Council for about six months, attempting to develop a national health insurance proposal for the Bush administration. Despite developing an interesting plan, reactionary elements within the White House ensured that it went nowhere. I have been a long-term advocate of an economically responsible national health insurance plan, and I was convinced that this would be a major issue for the 1992 election. This, in fact, proved to be true, and our failure to propose a credible national health insurance plan did not help the president's prospects for reelection (though the economic recession also did not help our campaign).

At the time of the election, I was working for a research consulting firm and volunteering as part of a group of senior advisers to the campaign. I remember well being assembled every other week with the other senior advisers for reasons that few of us were able to ascertain at the time. They never sought our advice, only our approval of ideas and commercials that would do little for the president's chances for reelection. In a six-month period, the president's approval numbers plummeted, with the campaign in denial until it was too late to recover the loss. I remember well the sad party in the Old Executive Office Building on the night of the election. As a result of the campaign's unwillingness to listen to what the public was saying, the country would be subject to eight years of the end-justifies-the-means politics of Bill Clinton, which did more to increase the nation's cynicism of any president since Richard Nixon.

Like most Americans, I actually liked Clinton on a personal level. Although I had only met him once very briefly, I had the impression that many have after meeting him personally or even seeing him interact with people on TV— that he would probably be fun to have a drink with. He also had the gift of overwhelming charisma that I had only witnessed once before, when I had the honor of meeting Ronald Reagan in 1991 in his Los Angeles office, after his presidency and before public disclosure of his illness. Although I was not a fan of the Reagan administration, and I was prepared to disagree with much of what he had to say, I found myself with a big smile on my face, glowing in the almost visible halo of this remarkable man's charisma. The same could be said about Bill Clinton, though to a somewhat lesser extent.

Unfortunately, Clinton squandered away this advantage, and whatever mandate he may have had from the election, with his various character flaws, particularly his almost pathological inability to tell the truth. By this time, I was working for Senator John McCain of Arizona. I spent over two years helping to beat down the National Health Security Act, the Clinton administration's humongous national health insurance plan, and trying to replace it with sound, economically responsible legislation. McCain did not oppose the Clinton plan because it was a Democratic plan; he opposed it because it was bad legislation at many different levels. The bill was developed in secret in an illegal manner and fundamentally reorganized the health care system in a manner that nobody could fully comprehend. No serious effort was made to accommodate the concerns of Republicans. I am proud to this day of my very small role in defeating the Clinton plan, though I would have strongly preferred if we had developed and enacted a good bill. I was also disturbed that many Republican senators would have attempted to defeat any such legislation on purely partisan political grounds.

During my time working for Senator McCain, I developed an enormous admiration for this man who, after spending five and a half years in a Vietnamese prison camp, rose up to become one of the most influential and publicly popular members of the US Senate. He made me realize that it is possible for politicians to attempt to do the right thing for our country irrespective of the demands of his party. While remaining a loyal member of the Republican Party for his entire life, he also demonstrated strong independence on some key issues against his party's positions: campaign finance reform, pork barrel spending, and the right to sue managed care plans, to mention a few. He paid a large political price for such independence during the 2000 presidential election, when the Republican Party insiders ensured that he would lose the nomination to the infinitely less qualified and less popular, but more willing to tow the conservative party line, George W. Bush.

Some will immediately dismiss this book as the sour grapes of a McCain supporter who cannot get past the defeat of his candidate. They would be correct to some extent, in that I maintain my outrage that a small group of Republican insiders was able, through untoward practices, to limit the Republican choice of all Americans to George W. Bush—a person of very modest talents who had never achieved anything on his own in his life without the assistance of family wealth and privilege, who had never even mustered the curiosity about other peoples and cultures to visit another country, and whose only qualification to be president was that his father had held the position. I am equally outraged that a small group of Democratic insiders was similarly able to limit our choice to Al Gore, a well-meaning politician of limited ability and almost no charisma whatsoever.

This book, therefore, will be characterized by partisans as the rantings of an angry and bitter person, and could be ignored as such except for two things. First, I am angry but not at all bitter; I like to characterize myself as a pessimistic optimist who believes our system will improve despite the best efforts of political partisans to impede progress. From my perspective, as only a slight overgeneralization, we have evolved from a situation of nobody at the wheel under Carter, to somebody at the wheel driving quickly, and sometimes erratically, in right and wrong directions under Reagan, to somebody at the wheel driving in basically the right direction but too slowly under Bush Sr., to someone driving in basically the right direction and speed but lying to us throughout the trip under Clinton, to someone with no business driving at all under George W. Bush. Still, we continue to survive, largely due to the collective wisdom of the American public and its affinity for divided government.

Second, while Americans do not necessarily share my views on our presidents, the majority of the American public shares my views of our two-party system. Surveys indicate that only about 25 percent of Americans believe that this system will solve the problems of our nation. To the greatest extent ever, Americans are seeking alternatives to Democratic and Republican candidates and are voting for political gridlock.

Some will see the title of this book and conclude that I am one of the "crazy conspiracy theorists" who perceive indictable offenses lurking in every corridor of Washington, DC. I do not fall in that category. In carefully choosing the term "conspiracy" to describe the behavior of the two major parties, I am not alleging a criminal conspiracy, though I would not rule anything out as impossible after some of the things we have seen in Washington in recent years. Rather, I am focusing on a much more subtle dynamic, whereby the two parties, which have a virtual oligopoly over our public policy, have colluded together in a legal manner to benefit themselves first and foremost. Sometimes this pursuit of mutual party interest has accrued to the benefit of the nation; more often, it has not.

This is not a kiss-and-tell book. With only a couple of exceptions, I have only the highest praise for everyone I worked with during my thirteen years in Washington. The problem is not fundamentally with the people who run our government; it is with the party-dominated system under which they operate. I have written this book because, after all these years, I remain an idealist. I believe the American public deserves better than the constant "least common denominator" approaches and "lesser of evils" choices that are presented to us. We deserve better than the legalized political corruption that has been "legitimized" by the political process, but continues to fuel the cynicism that pervades our political system. We deserve better than the vote trading, "you scratch my back and I'll scratch yours" mentality that remains the worst of our political heritage. We deserve an end of the two-party Democratic-Republican conspiracy against the American public.

Andrew I. Batavia
Associate Professor
Florida International University

Appendix F.
Lifetime Checklist

Drew was always planning ahead. This lifetime checklist was found on Drew's hard drive after his death. Some of these goals had already been accomplished: AUTONOMY, Inc.; the independent living book. Others were planned. We can now check "Memoir" off his list.

Joseph
Katey
Panama Canal
Israel
Russia
Vietnam
Rhine cruise
US road trip
Memoir
Bull Moose Reform Party
AUTONOMY, Inc.
Independent living book
Political book
International book
China
Europe
Screenplay

Appendix G.
Curriculum Vitae

A listing of Drew's education, research/scholarship, teaching, service, and honors is included below. Much of his employment history can be found in his memoirs and a timeline (Appendix A). The style used for Florida International University tenure application was maintained.

ANDREW I. BATAVIA

EDUCATION

1980-1982 HARVARD LAW SCHOOL, J.D., June 1984

1983-1984 STANFORD LAW SCHOOL (non-matriculating student status)

1982-1983 STANFORD UNIVERSITY MEDICAL SCHOOL, M.S. in Health Services Research, October 1983 (Took leave of absence from Harvard)

1976-1980 UNIVERSITY OF CALIFORNIA, Riverside, B.A., Economics and Sociology, June 1980

1975-1976 UNIVERSITY OF CALIFORNIA, Berkeley

RESEARCH AND SCHOLARSHIP

Books

Batavia, A.I. *Independent Living: A Viable Option for Long-Term Care,* ABI Professional Publications, Clearwater, FL, 2003.

Batavia, A.I. 1990. *Meeting the Health Care Needs of Physically Disabled Persons in the Netherlands: Implications for U.S. Policy*, New York: Rehabilitation International.

Batavia, A.I. 1988. *The Payment of Medical Rehabilitation Services: Current Mechanisms and Potential Models*, Chicago, IL: American Hospital Association.

Papers in Professional Journals

Articles

Articles in Law Journals

Batavia, A.I. "Disability Rights in the Third Stage of the Independent Living Movement," *Stanford Journal of Law and Policy* (in press).

Batavia, A.I. "The Growing Prominence of Independent Living and Consumer Direction as Principles in Long-Term Care: A Content Analysis," *Elder Law Journal* (in press).

Batavia, A.I. 2002. "Disability vs. Futility in Rationing Health Care Services: Defining Medical Futility Based on Permanent Unconsciousness – PVS, Coma and Anencephaly," *Behavioral Sciences and the Law* 20: 219-33.

Batavia, A.I. 2001. "A Right to Personal Assistance Services: 'Most Integrated Setting Appropriate' Requirements and the Independent Living Model of Long-Term Care," *American Journal of Law and Medicine* 27(1): 17-43.

Batavia, A.I. 2000. "So Far, So Good: Observations on the First Year of the Oregon Death with Dignity Act," in Special Theme Issue: Hastened Death, G. Andrew H. Benjamin, James L. Werth, Jr. & Lawrence Gostin (eds.), *Psychology, Public Policy and Law* 6(2): 291-305.

Batavia, A.I. 2000. "The Relevance of Physician and Disability Data on the Right to Physician-Assisted Suicide: Can Studies Resolve the Issue?," in Special Theme Issue: Hastened Death, G. Andrew H. Benjamin, James L. Werth, Jr. & Lawrence Gostin (eds.), *Psychology, Public Policy and Law* 6(2): 546-558.

Batavia, A.I., G. DeJong, and L. McKnew. 1991. "Toward a National Personal Assistance Program: The Independent Living Model of Long-Term Care for Persons with Disabilities," *Journal of Health Politics, Policy and Law* 16(3): 523-545.

Batavia, A.I. 1984. "Preferred Provider Organizations: Antitrust Aspects and Implications for the Hospital Industry," *American Journal of Law and Medicine* 10(2): 169-188, Summer 1984.

Batavia, A.I. 1983. "Blue Cross-Blue Shield Payment Policies: Antitrust Aspects and Implications for the Health Care and Insurance Industries," *National Federation of Insurance Counsel Quarterly* 33(2): 173-212, Winter 1983.

Articles in Refereed Journals

Batavia, A.I. "Managed Care and Independent Living," *Journal of Rehabilitation Educators* (in press).

Batavia, A.I. 2003. "Accounting for the health-care bill," Lancet 362 number 9394, 1495-1497.

Batavia, A.I. 2002. "Consumer Direction, Consumer Choice and the Future of Long-Term Care," *Journal of Disability Policy Studies* 13(2): 67-73, 86.

Batavia, A.I. and Schriner, K. 2001. "The ADA as Engine of Social Change: The Strengths and Limitations of a Civil Rights Approach to Meeting the Needs of People with Disabilities," *Policy Studies Journal*, 29(4): 690-702.

Schriner, K. and Batavia, A.I., 2001. "The Americans with Disabilities Act: Does It Secure the Fundamental Right to Vote?," *Policy Studies Journal*, 29(4): 663-73.

Batavia, A.I. 2001. "The Ethics of PAS: Morally Relevant Relationships Between Personal Assistance Services and

Physician-Assisted Suicide." *Archives of Physical Medicine and Rehabilitation*, 2001;12 Suppl 2:S25-31.

Batavia, A.I. 2001. "Are People with Disabilities an Oppressed Minority, and Why Does This Matter?" in (Batavia, AI, guest editor) Special Issue on Oppression and Disability, *Journal of Disability Policy Studies*, 12(2): 66-67 (Fall 2001).

Batavia, A.I. 2001. "The New Paternalism: Characterizing People with Disabilities as an Oppressed Minority," in (Batavia, AI, guest editor) Special Issue on Oppression and Disability, *Journal of Disability Policy Studies*, 12(2): 107-13 (Fall 2001).

Batavia, M., Batavia, A.I, and Friedman, R. 2001. "Changing Chairs: Anticipating Problems in Prescribing Wheelchairs." *Disability and Rehabilitation* 23(12): 539-48.

Batavia, A.I. and DeJong, G. 2001. "Disability, Chronic Illness and Risk Selection," *Archives of Physical Medicine and Rehabilitation*, 81: 546-52 (April 2001).

Batavia, A.I. and Beaulaurier, R. 2001. "The Financial Vulnerability of People with Disabilities: Assessing Poverty Risks." *Sociology and Social Welfare* March 2001, 28(1): 139-62.

Batavia, A.I. 1999. "Of Wheelchairs and Managed Care." *Health Affairs* 18(6): 177-82 (November/December 1999).

Batavia, A.I. 1999. "Independent Living Centers, Medical Rehabilitation Centers, and Managed Health Care for People with Disabilities." *Archives of Physical Medicine and Rehabilitation*, 80 (October 1999): 1357-60.

Batavia, M. and Batavia, A.I. 1999. "Pressure Ulcer in Man with Tetraplegia and a Poorly Fitting Wheelchair: A Case Report with Clinical and Policy Implications." *Spinal Cord* (1999) 37: 140-41.

Batavia, A.I. 1998. "The Prospects for a National Personal Assistance Services Program for People With Disabilities," *American Rehabilitation*," 24 (3), Winter 1998.

Batavia, A.I. 1997. "Disability and Physician-Assisted Suicide." *The New England Journal of Medicine*, 336(23): 1671-73, June 5, 1997.

Batavia, A.I. 1997. "Ideology and the Independent Living Movement: Will Conservatism Harm People with Disabilities?" *The Annals of the American Academy of Political and Social Science*, 549: 10-23, January 1997.

Batavia, A.I., and S. Parker. 1995. "From Disability Rolls to Payrolls: A Proposal for Social Security Program Reform," *Journal of Disability Policy Studies* 6(1): 73-86, August 1995.

Batavia, A.I., R. Ozminkowski, G. Gaumer and M. Gabay. 1994. "Lessons for States in Inpatient Ratesetting Under the Boren Amendment," *Health Care Financing Review* 15(2): 137-54.

Batavia, A.I. 1993. "Relating Disability Policy to Broader Public Policy: Understanding the Concept of Handicap," *Policy Studies Journal*. 21(4): 735-39.

Batavia, A.I. 1993. "Health Care Reform and People With Disabilities," *Health Affairs* 12(1): 40-57, Spring 1993.

Batavia, A.I. 1992. "Assessing the Function of Functional Assessment: A Consumer Perspective," *Disability and Rehabilitation* 14(3): 156-160.

DeJong, G., A.I. Batavia, and L. McKnew. 1992. "The Independent Living Model of Personal Assistance in National Long-Term-Care Policy," *Generations* Winter 1992: 89-95. Reprinted in *Aging and Disabilities: Seeking Common Ground* (E.F. Ansello and N.F. Eustis, Eds.), New York: Baywood Publishing Co., 1993.

Wilkerson, D., A.I. Batavia, and G. DeJong. 1992. "The Use of Functional Status Measures for Payment of Medical Rehabilitation Services." *Archives of Physical Medicine and Rehabilitation* 73: 111-20, February 1992.

Batavia, A.I., G. DeJong, and L. McKnew. 1991. "Toward a National Personal Assistance Program: The Independent Living Model of Long-Term Care for Persons with Disabilities," *Journal of Health Politics, Policy and Law* 16(3): 523-545.

Burns, T.J., A.I. Batavia, and G. DeJong. 1991. "The Health Insurance Coverage of Working-Age Persons with Physical Disabilities," *Inquiry* 28(2): 187-93, Summer 1991.

DeJong, G., and A.I. Batavia. 1991. "Toward a Health Services Research Capacity in Spinal Cord Injury," *Paraplegia* 29: 373-89, Summer 1991. Reprinted in *Management of Spinal Cord Injury*, Second Edition (C.P. Zejdlik, ed.), Boston: Jones and Bartlett, 1992.

Batavia, A.I. 1991. "A Disability Rights/Independent Living Perspective on Euthanasia," *The Western Journal of Medicine* 154: 616-17, May 1991.

Batavia, A.I., and G. Hammer. 1991. "Toward the Development of Consumer-Based Criteria for the Evaluation of Assistive Devices," *Journal of Rehabilitation Research and Development*, 27(4): 425-36, 1991.

DeJong, G., and A.I. Batavia. 1990. "The Americans With Disabilities Act and the Current State of Disability Policy," *Journal of Disability Policy Studies*, 1(3): 65-75, Fall 1990.

Batavia, A.I., G. DeJong, E.A. Eckenhoff, and R.S. Materson. 1990. "After the Americans With Disabilities Act: The Role of the Rehabilitation Community." *Archives of Physical Medicine and Rehabilitation* 71(12): 1014-15, Nov. 1990.

Batavia, A.I., and G. DeJong. 1990. "Developing a Comprehensive Health Services Research Capacity in Physical Disability and Rehabilitation," *Journal of Disability Policy Studies*, 1(1): 37-61, Spring 1990.

DeJong, G., A.I. Batavia, and J.M. Williams. 1990. "Who is Responsible for the Lifelong Well-Being of a Person With a Head Injury?" *Journal of Head Trauma Rehabilitation*, 5(1): 9-22, March 1990. Reprinted in *The Psychological and Social*

Impact of Disability (Marinelli, R.P. and A.E. Del Orto, Eds.), N.Y.: Springer Publishing Co.

Burns, T.J., A.I. Batavia, Q.W. Smith, and G. DeJong. 1990. "The Primary Health Care Needs of Persons With Physical Disabilities: What Are The Research and Service Priorities?," *Archives of Physical Medicine and Rehabilitation*, 71(2): 138-143, 1990.

DeJong, G., A.I. Batavia, and R. Griss. 1989. "America's Neglected Health Minority: Working-Age Persons with Disabilities." *The Milbank Quarterly*, 67 (Supplement 2, Part 2): 311-351.

Batavia, A.I. 1989. "Representation and Role Separation in the Disability Movement: Should Researchers Be Advocates?" *Archives of Physical Medicine and Rehabilitation*, 70(4): 345-348, April 1989.

DeJong, G., and A.I. Batavia. 1989. "Societal Duty and Resource Allocation For Persons With Severe Traumatic Brain Injury," *Journal of Head Trauma Rehabilitation*, 4(1): 1-12, March 1989.

Batavia, A.I,, G. DeJong, L.S. Halstead, and Q.W. Smith. 1988. "Primary Medical Services for People With Disabilities," *American Rehabilitation*, 14(4): 9-12, 26-27, Winter 1988.

Batavia, A.I. and G. DeJong. 1988. "Prospective Payment for Medical Rehabilitation: The DHHS Report to Congress," *Archives of Physical Medicine and Rehabilitation* 69(5): 377-380, May 1988.

Proceedings

Batavia, A.I. 1998. Comments by Andrew I. Batavia in "Conference: Socially-Assisted Dying: Media, Money and Meaning," *Cornell Journal of Law and Public Policy*, 7(2): 273-78, 292-93, 348-49, 394-963, Winter 1998.

Batavia, A.I. and G. Hammer. 1989. "Consumer Criteria for Evaluating Assistive Devices: Implications for Technology Transfer," Proceedings of the 12th Annual Conference of the Rehabilitation Engineering Society of North America, June 1989.

Chapters in Books

Batavia, A.I. "'Sure I Want to Work–That's the Ticket': Disability, Human Nature and the Ticket-to-Work Program," in *[title of book to be determined]*, K. Rupp and S. Bell, (eds.), Washington, D.C.: Urban Institute Press (in press).

Batavia, A.I. 2000. "Ten Years Later: The Americans With Disabilities Act and the Future of Disability Policy," in L. Francis and A. Silvers (ed.), *Americans with Disabilities: Exploring the Implications of the Law for Individuals and Institutions*, New York: Routledge Press, 283-292.

Batavia, A.I. 1998. "Unsustainable Growth: Preserving Disability Programs for Americans with Disabilities," in *Growth in Disability Benefits: Explanations and Policy Implications*, K. Rupp and D. Stapleton, (eds.), Kalamazoo, MI: W.E. Upjohn Institute for Employment Research, 1998: 325-36.

Batavia, A.I. 1996. "Health Care, Personal Assistance, and Assistive Technology: Are In-Kind Benefits Key to Independence or Dependence for People with Disabilities?," In *Disability, Cash Benefits and Work,* J.L. Mashaw, et al., (eds.), Kalamazoo, MI: W.E. Upjohn Institute for Employment Research.

Batavia, A.I. 1996. "Public Accommodations" in *Implementing the Americans with Disabilities Act,* West, J. (ed.), Cambridge, MA: Milbank Memorial Fund, Blackwell Publishers, Inc.

Schriner, K.F.and A.I. Batavia. 1995. "Disability, Law and Social Policy" in *Encyclopedia Of Disability* (A.E. Dell Orto and R.P. Marinelli, Editors); New York: Simon & Schuster Macmillan.

Government Reports or Monographs
(provided editing, but not authorship)

National Academy on Aging, *Advisory Panel Report on the Future of Community-Based Long-Term Care.* 1994. (Served as member of the advisory panel), The Maxwell School of Citizenship and Public Affairs, Syracuse University, Syracuse, New York, October 1994.

National Council on Disability. 1993. (Batavia, A.I., Executive Director) *ADA Watch: Year One—Report to the President and the Congress on Progress in Implementing the Americans with Disabilities Act,* Washington, DC: NCD, April 1993.

National Council on Disability. 1993. (Batavia, A.I., Executive Director) *Meeting the Unique Needs of Minorities With Disabilities—A Report to the President and the Congress*, Washington, DC: NCD, April 26, 1993.

National Council on Disability. 1993. (Batavia, A.I., Executive Director) *Annual Report to the President and the Congress, Volume 13—Fiscal Year 1992*, Washington, DC: NCD, March 30, 1993.

National Council on Disability. 1993. (Batavia, A.I., Executive Director) *Sharing the Risk and Ensuring Independence: A Disability Perspective on Access to Health Insurance and Health-Related Services—A Report to the President and the Congress*, Washington, DC: NCD, March 4.

National Council on Disability. 1993. (Batavia, A.I., Executive Director) *Study on the Financing of Assistive Technology and Services for Individuals with Disabilities—A Report to the President and the Congress*, Washington, DC: NCD, March 4, 1993.

National Council on Disability. 1993. (Batavia, A.I., Executive Director) *Serving the Nation's Students with Disabilities: Progress and Prospects—A Report to the President and the Congress*, Washington, DC: NCD, March 4, 1993.

OTHER PUBLICATIONS

Batavia, A.I. 1989. *The Legal Liability of Independent Living Centers*, Houston, Texas: Independent Living Resource Utilization (ILRU), July 1989.

Articles

Batavia, A.I. and G. DeJong. 1990. "The Language of Disability Policy: A Matter of Semantics?" *Journal of Disability Policy Studies* 1(4): 1990.

Batavia, A.I. 1988. "Needed: Active Therapeutic Recreation for High Level Quadriplegics," *Therapeutic Recreation Journal*, 22(2): 8-11, Second Quarter 1988.

Proceedings

Batavia, A.I., D. Dillard, and B. Phillips. 1990. "How to Avoid Technology Abandonment," Proceedings of the Fifth Annual Conference on Technology and Persons with Disabilities (ed. Harry Murphy), Los Angeles, CA, California State University at Northridge, March 21-24, 1990.

Chapters

Burns, T.J., A.I. Batavia and G. DeJong. 1994. "The Health Insurance Work Disincentive for People with Disabilities," in *Research in the Sociology of Health Care, Volume II*, JAI Press: Greenwich, Connecticut, 1994.

DeJong, G., R.W. Brannon, and A.I. Batavia. 1993. "Financing Health and Personal Care" in *Aging With a Spinal Cord Injury* (eds. Whiteneck, G.G. et al), New York: Demos Publications.

Book Reviews

Batavia, A.I. 1999. "Book Review—Rethinking Health Care Policy: The New Politics of State Regulation by Robert Hackey." 35 *Inquiry* 449 (Winter 1998-99).

Batavia, A.I. 1998. "Book Review—Blackbird Fly Away: Disabled in an Able-Bodied World by Hugh Gregory Gallagher." *Journal of Disability Policy Studies*.

Non-Refereed Journal Articles

Radensky P.W., Zimmerman E.P., Batavia A.I. 1997. "Changing practice expense values: impact on radiology payment." *Radiology Management.* 1997 Jan-Feb;19(1):12-3, 15-7.

Radensky, P.W. and Batavia, A.I. 1997. "Balancing Cost and Outcomes," *Health Measures*, January 1997.

Millman D.S., Zimmerman E.P., Batavia A.I., Radensky P.W. 1996. "HCFA's Correct Coding Initiative: implications for radiology." *Radiology Management,* 1996 Nov-Dec;18(5):14, 16-8.

Radensky, P.W. and Batavia, A.I. 1996. "Low-Osmolar Contrast Media: Current Markets, Future Prospects," *Imaging Economics*.

Newspaper Articles

Batavia, A.I. 2001. "Ashcroft and Oregon's Death with Dignity Act: Action threatens the GOP" *The Miami Herald*, Page 7B, December 11, 2001.

Batavia, A.I. 1997. "New gadgets allow wheelchairs to have access to beach" *The Miami Herald*, Page 2C, July 29, 1997.

Batavia, A.I. 1997. "Law aims to balance needs of schools with disabled students' rights" *The Miami Herald*, Page 2C, June 3, 1997.

Batavia, A.I. 1997. "Legal aliens who pay taxes, do fair share are entitled to benefits" *The Miami Herald*, Page 2C, May 20, 1997.

Batavia, A.I. 1997. "Flat tax could claim larger slice of income of disabled people" *The Miami Herald*, Page 2C, May 6, 1997.

Batavia, A.I. 1997. "Should disabled people support a legal right to doctor-assisted suicide?" *The Miami Herald*, Page 2C, April 22, 1997.

Batavia, A.I. 1997. "Should FDR's disability be visually depicted on his memorial?" *The Miami Herald*, Page 2C, February 25, 1997.

McCain, John. 1994. "Political Autopsy: Clinton Administration's 'Malpractice' Killed Health Care Reform." *Mesa Tribune,* A13, October 14, 1994.

McCain, John. 1994. "Mitchell Health Bill Just a Clinton Rehash." *Arizona Republic,* C3, August 14, 1994.

McCain, John. 1994. "Health Reform: A Battle of Opposing Visions." *Phoenix Gazette* (Opinions B7), April 21, 1994.

McCain, John. 1993. "Alternative Approach: Health Care Reform Should Adhere to Tenets of Free Market." *Mesa Tribune* (Perspective, Section J), November 28, 1993.

McCain, John. 1993. "Clinton's Cure Worse Than the Disease." *Arizona Republic,* B7, October 13, 1993.

"The Netherlands Health Care System and People with Physical Disabilities—An Interview with Andrew Batavia," *International Rehabilitation Review* XLI(2 & 3): IDEAS Portfolio II (p. 14-15).

Letters to the Editor, Progress Reports, Etc.

Batavia, A.I. 2002. "If They Are So Smart, They Should Start Their Own School," *New Times,* September 2002 (Letter to the editor).

Batavia, A.I. 2002. "For Autonomy in Life and Death." *The Oregonian,* April 23, 2002 (Letter to the Editor).

Batavia, A.I. 2001. "A Call for Civility in the Disability/Assisted Suicide Debate," *Psychology, Public Policy and Law* 7(3): 728 (Letter to the editor).

Batavia, A.I. 2001. "Don't Use Scare Tactics in Assisted Death Debate," *Times Union*, March 30, 2001 (Letter to the editor).

Batavia, A.I., and K. Schriner. 1998. "Disability, Oppression & Autonomy: A Call for Papers for a Special Issue of the JDPS?," *Journal of Disability Policy Studies* 9(1): 1-5, 1998.

DeJong, G., A.I. Batavia, T.J. Burns, G. Markert, and M. Meehan. 1990. "Health Insurance-Related Work Disincentives for SSDI Beneficiaries," *Rehabilitation R & D Progress Reports 1989* (26)1: 469, February 1990.

Batavia, A.I. and G. Hammer. 1990. "Developing Consumer Criteria for Evaluating Assistive Devices," *Rehabilitation R & D Progress Reports 1989* (26)1: 464-65, February 1990.

Batavia, A.I. 1990. "Primary Care for Persons with Disabilities in the Netherlands," *Rehabilitation R & D Progress Reports 1989* (26)1: 465-66, February 1990.

Naierman, N., R. Brannon, A.I. Batavia, and G. DeJong. 1990. "A Managed Primary Health Care Program for Working-Age Persons with Physical Disabilities—Planning for Implementation," *Rehabilitation R & D Progress Reports 1989* (26)1: 468, February 1990.

DeJong, G., A.I. Batavia, T.J. Burns, and S.E. Melus. 1989. "Delphi Survey and National Invitational Conference on the

Primary Health Care Needs of Persons with Physical Disabilities," *Rehabilitation R & D Progress Reports 1988*, 25(1): 374-74, January 1989.

DeJong, G., and A.I. Batavia. 1989. "A Capitation-Financed Managed Health Care Program for Working-Age Persons with Severe Disabilities," *Rehabilitation R & D Progress Reports 1988*, 25(1): 375-76, January 1989.

Batavia, A.I. 1988. "The Finance of Medical Rehabilitation Services: Interim Report on the Mary E. Switzer Distinguished Research Fellowship in Medical Rehabilitation Finance," *Rehabilitation R & D Progress Reports 1987*, 25(1): 451-52, January 1988.

Batavia, A.I. 1987. "Blowdarts," *Paraplegia News* 41(10):43, (October 1987); reprinted in *Sports 'n Spokes* 13(4): 47, November 1987.

Batavia, A.I. 1983. *Prospects and Strategies for the Teaching Hospital Under Medicare DRG Reimbursement*, Master's thesis available through Stanford University Library, December 1983.

Batavia, A.I. 1979. "The Finance of the Swedish Health Care System," *The Dialectic* (academic journal of U.C. Riverside), 1979.

PRESENTED PAPERS

Throughout my career, I have spoken before a wide variety of different audiences. These were all invited presentations. Most of these conferences were held by prominent national organizations. In all cases in which substantial travel was required, all travel expenses for me and my personal assistant, who must accompany me due to my disability, were paid by the organization. This has allowed me to allocate whatever travel funds have been available through FIU to a junior colleague who needed the funds. I believe such invitations from national organizations are evidence of respect for my work and expertise in the field. The following is a list of my presentations:[1]

Speaker, will present "Ethical Issues and Spinal Cord Injury," in the Annual Conference of the American Society on Spinal Cord Injury, in Bal Harbour, May 2003.

Speaker, presented "Death on Your Own Terms," in the Annual Conference of the South Florida Model Spinal Cord Injury System, held at the Miami Project, Jackson Memorial Medical Center, University of Miami School of Medicine, September 27, 2002.

Speaker, presented commentary for the "Ticket-to-Work Conference," sponsored by The Social Security Administration and the Urban Institute, Washington, DC, May 2002.

Speaker, presented "Models of Long-term Care for People with Disabilities," in the Switzer Research Fellowship Seminar sponsored by the National Institute on Disability and Rehabilitation Research, Arlington, VA, May 2002.

Panel Member, "Independent Choices Symposium," sponsored by the Office on Disability, Aging & Long-Term

Care Policy, DHHS, L'Enfant Plaza Hotel, Washington, DC, June 10-12, 2001.

Panel Member, "Disability Income Policy: Opportunities and Challenges in the Next Decade—A Policy Education Seminar, sponsored by the Social Security Administration and the National Academy of Social Insurance. Washington Court Hotel, Washington, DC, December 15, 2000.

Panel Member, "Consumer Choice for Disabled Beneficiaries Under Medicare," sponsored by the Health Insurance Reform Project. Governor's House Hotel, Washington, DC, September 21-22, 2000.

Speaker, NIDRR Summer 2000 Researcher's Symposium on Qualitative Research. Presented "Issues of Generalizability and Impact: Advocacy, Qualitative Research, and Bias in the Policy Process." University of Iowa, Iowa City, July 28, 2000.

Speaker, California Conference on Assisted Dying. Presented "The View from the Slippery Slope: People with Disabilities and Physician-Assisted Suicide." University of California, San Francisco, November 13, 1998.

Speaker, Conference on "The Affirmative Action Seesaw: Mend It—End It—Then What?," sponsored by the University of Miami, the Business Coalition for Americans with Disabilities, and the Office of Federal Contract Compliance Programs. Miami Airport Hilton Towers, March 26, 1998.

Speaker, "Conference on Socially Assisted Dying," sponsored by the Rehabilitation Institution of Chicago and Northwestern University. Chicago, IL, April 12-13, 1997.

Luncheon Keynote Speaker, "Issues in the Media: End of Life Issues," sponsored by the American Medical Association. New York, NY, April 18, 1997.

Luncheon Keynote Speaker, California Leadership Association. Riverside, CA, May 1997.

Panel Member, Presented comments on the policy implications panel of the SSA/Lewin-VHI conference on the "Social Security Administration's Disability Programs: Explanations of Recent Growth and Implications for Disability Policy." Washington, DC, July 21, 1995.

Commencement Speaker, Delivered the commencement address at the University of California, Riverside, graduation. Riverside, CA, June 17, 1995.

Speaker, "People with Disabilities as a Vulnerable Population" at a meeting of the National Health Policy Forum. Washington, DC, December 7, 1995.

Speaker, Presented "In-Kind Benefits: Key to Independence or Dependence for People with Disabilities" at a conference of the National Academy of Social Insurance. Santa Monica, CA, December 8-10, 1994.

Speaker, Presented "Research Issues Concerning Policy on Assistive Technology" at a meeting of the Office of

Disability, Aging and Long-term Care Policy, DHHS. Washington, DC, November 10, 1994.

Speaker and Panel Member, Session II on "Putting Research to Work for the Realization of the ADA: The Perspective of the Disability Community," National Council on Disability Conference on "Furthering the Goals of the ADA Through Disability Policy Research in the 1990s," December 7-9, 1992. Presented "The Failure of Disability Policy Research: Sources and Solutions." Washington, DC, December 7, 1992.

Featured Participant, "A Conversation With Andrew Batavia," sponsored by the American Public Health Association, Disablement Caucus. Washington, DC, November 10, 1992.

Panel Member, "Health Care Financing Issues" and "Health Care Delivery Issues," American Speech Language Hearing Association Annual Conference. Washington, DC, June 1992.

Keynote Speaker, "Five Basic Questions for Disability Researchers: Reconsidering Why, Who, What, How, and Where," Mary E. Switzer Commemorative Rehabilitation Research Seminar, sponsored by NIDRR. Washington, DC, April 13, 1992.

Keynote Speaker, "Future Trends in Program Eligibility and Benefits: The Use of Functional Assessment," National Institutes of Health Conference on Diagnosis of Neuromuscular Disease. Bethesda, MD, March 11, 1992.

Speaker, "Topics in Health Policy," HSR Seminar Series, Stanford University Medical School. Stanford, CA, October 1, 1991.

Panel Member, "Who Lives, Who Dies: Technological Advances and Ethical Choices," Stanford University Centennial Roundtable. Stanford, CA, September 31, 1991.

Panel Member, "Functional Assessment in Health Care Facilities," National Health Policy Forum. Washington, DC, May 1, 1991.

Master of Ceremonies, "The Future is Now: Employing Persons with Disabilities at DOJ and Beyond," Department of Justice Observance of National Disability Employment Awareness Month. Washington, DC, October 30, 1990.

Participant, Meeting of the Centers for Disease Control (CDC) Committee on Injury Prevention. Atlanta, GA, August 30, 1990.

Participant, Meeting of the NIH Task Force on Medical Rehabilitation Research. Hunt Valley, MD, June 28-29, 1990.

Panel Member, Medlantic Fifth Annual Bioethics Seminar— Dialogue on Death and Dying: Panel on "Ethics of Choice: Putting Limits on Health Care." Washington, DC, June 14, 1990.

Speaker, SCI Model Systems Annual Conference, Presented "Implications of the Current SCI Knowledge Database." Washington, DC, December 1989.

Participant, Brookings Institute Conference on Long-Term Care for the Non-elderly Population. Washington, DC, July 1989.

Speaker, Twelfth Annual Conference of RESNA (Rehabilitation Engineering Society of North America), June 25-30, 1989: Presented "Consumer Criteria for Evaluating Assistive Devices: Implications for Technology Transfer." New Orleans, LA, June 26, 1989.

Speaker, Twenty-Ninth Law Institute on Hospitals and Physicians, Presented "The Financing of Medical Rehabilitation Hospitals and Units: Implications for the Health Care Industry." Richmond, VA, March 24, 1989.

Participant, Electronic Industries Foundation's Rehabilitation Engineering Center Invitational Conference, "Workshop on Implementing Technology Utilization." Washington, DC, March 8-10, 1989.

Speaker, American Congress of Rehabilitation Medicine Annual Conference, Seattle, October 28-November 5, 1988: Presented "Disability and Health Policy: The Disabled Person as a Consumer of Health Care Services." October 29, 1988.

Speaker, Rehabilitation Hospital Services Corporation Annual Conference, Presented "The Future of Medical Rehabilitation Financing," Washington, DC, October 17, 1988.

Speaker, NRH National Invitational Conference on the Primary Health Care Needs of Persons With Physical Disabilities, September 28-29, 1988: Presented with Gerben

DeJong, Ph.D. "The Results of NRH's Managed Health Care Feasibility Study Sponsored by The Robert Wood Johnson Foundation." Washington, DC, Sept. 29, 1988.

Speaker, National Rehabilitation Caucus Steering Committee Meeting, "Results of the Mary E. Switzer Distinguished Research Fellowship in Rehabilitation Finance." Washington, DC, August 12, 1988.

Speaker, National Association of Rehabilitation Facilities Annual Conference on "Waves of the Future," Puerto Rico, June 16-19, 1988: Presented "The Financing of Medical Rehabilitation Services: The 1990s and Beyond." Rio Grande, Puerto Rico, June 17, 1988.

Speaker and Participant, National Institute on Disability and Rehabilitation Research Invitational Conference, "Working Group Meeting on Health Insurance Practices and Policies Which Affect Individuals With Disabilities." Washington, DC, June 14-15, 1988.

Speaker, National Rehabilitation Hospital Research Seminar: Presented "The Future of Rehabilitation Financing: Implications for the Rehabilitation Hospital." Washington, DC, June 9, 1988.

Participant, American Association for the Advancement of Science National Invitational Conference, "Workshop on the Demography of Scientists and Engineers With Disabilities," co-sponsored by the American Statistical Association. Washington, DC, January 29-30, 1988.

Faculty Member, American Hospital Association
Rehabilitation Hospital Section Annual Conference on "The
Economics of Rehabilitation," November 14-18, 1987:
Presented "Current Mechanisms and Potential Models for the
Payment of Medical Rehabilitation." Los Angeles, CA,
November 17, 1987.

WORKS IN PROGRESS

Papers submitted to journals for consideration

Batavia, M. and Batavia, A.I. "Medical Errors: Putting the
Patient in the Picture." Submitted to *The New England
Journal of Medicine*.

Batavia, A.I. "Physician-Assisted Suicide as an Autonomy-
Based Right: Getting Beyond the Rhetoric" in K. Kirshner
(ed.), Physician-Assisted Suicide: Disability Perspectives,
Northwestern University Press.

Batavia, A.I. "Accounting for the Health Care Bill."
Submitted to *Health Affairs*.

Batavia, A.I. and Batavia, M. "Karaoke for Quads: A
New Application of an Old Recreational Activity."
Submitted to *Disability and Rehabilitation*.

Other completed papers

Batavia, A.I. and Batavia, M. "Iatrogenic Illness,
Disability and Chronic Condition." Soon to be
submitted to *Archives of Physical Medicine and
Rehabilitation*.

Research in Progress

Batavia, A.I. "Medical Savings Accounts and People at High Risk of Health Problems" (in progress).

Batavia, A.I. "Medical Necessity and a Patient's Right to Sue: The Illusion of Objectivity and Fairness in Managed Care Rationing Decisions" (in progress).

Batavia, A.I. "Respiratory Failure and Respiratory Success" (in progress).

Batavia, A.I. and Batavia, M. "Disability, Chronic Condition and Iatrogenic Illness" (in progress).

b. Papers/Presentations at Meetings/Conferences

c. Exhibits, Shows, Recitals, Etc.

N.A.

d. Research Grants/Contracts

The following is a list of my grants and contracts over a period of approximately fifteen years. Unfortunately, I do not have title pages for these proposals. All of these grants were for relatively small amounts of money. As I indicated earlier, the type of theoretical, legal, and policy-oriented research I do typically does not attract large grant funding.

2001-2002   Distinguished Research Fellow, Mary E. Switzer Distinguished Research Fellowship,

U.S. Department of Education. "Fellowship on the Financing of the Long-Term Care Continuum." Research on different models of long-term care: the informal support model; the medical model; and the independent living model. $55,000.

1998-2000   Project Consultant, Research and Training Center on Managed Care and Disability funded by the National Institute on Disability and Rehabilitation Research. Developed paper on risk adjustment and disability. $3,000.

1998-1999   Project Consultant, "Cash and Counseling Demonstration and Evaluation Project," funded by the Robert Wood Johnson Foundation and the Office of the Assistant Secretary for Planning and Evaluation, U.S. Department of Health and Human Services. Assisted in addressing issues concerning the younger population of people with disabilities. $1,000.

1997-1998   Principal Investigator, "Independent Living Centers and Health Care for People with Disabilities," funded by Independent Living Research Utilization, Inc.: Conducted a survey of independent living centers to determine the extent to which they are addressing health care issues. $4,000. Final report is included in the publications section.

1992-1993   Project Consultant, "Constituency-Oriented Research and Evaluation," under a contract from NIDRR. Developed a policy on participation by NIDRR's constituencies in its research. $5,000.

1989-1990   Principal Investigator, "A National Invitational Conference on Developing a Comprehensive Health Services Research Capacity in Physical Disability and Rehabilitation," funded by NIDRR: Developed the first national invitational conference addressing issues concerning health services research and physical disability. $50,000. Final report is included in the publications section.

1989   International Fellow, "Approaches to Addressing the Primary Health Care Needs of Persons With Disabilities in the Netherlands," International Disability Exchanges and Studies (IDEAS) Program of World Institute of Disability (WID) and Rehabilitation International (RI), May-June 1989. $10,000. Final report is included in the publications section.

1988-1990   Principal Investigator, "A Managed Care Program for Working-Age Persons with Severe Physical Disabilities: Technical Design and Development Stage," funded by The Robert Wood Johnson Foundation and conducted at NRH: Designed a managed health care program for persons with physical disabilities in the Washington, DC, metropolitan area. $100,000. Final report is included in the publications section.

1988-1990   Principal Investigator, "Health Insurance Coverage of Disability Beneficiaries," funded by the Social Security Administration (SSA): Examined access to and adequacy of private health insurance benefits available to persons eligible for Medicare and/or Medicaid, and health insurance-related work disincentives for such individuals. $50,000. An article based on this study is included in the publications section.

1988-1989   Principal Investigator, "Consumer-Based Criteria for the Assessment of Rehabilitation Technologies: Toward a Theory of Evaluation for Rehabilitation Engineering," a research project of the NRH Rehabilitation Engineering Center in Evaluation funded by NIDRR: Examined the criteria used by persons with disabilities in adopting or abandoning assistive devices. $10,000. A published abstract and a peer-reviewed article on this study are included in the publications section.

1987-1988   Project Director, "A Capitation-Financed Managed Care Program for Persons with Severe Disabilities: A Feasibility Study," funded by the Robert Wood Johnson Foundation and conducted at NRH: Directed study on feasibility of developing a capitation financed managed health care program for persons with physical disabilities in the Washington, DC, metropolitan area. $100,000. Final report is included in the publications section.

1987-1988   Conference Director, "A National Invitational Conference on the Primary Health Care Needs of Persons With Physical Disabilities," funded by NIDRR and conducted by NRH, September 28-29, 1988: Directed the first national invitational conference addressing issues concerning the post-rehabilitation primary health care needs of the physically disabled population. $50,000. Final report is included in the publications section.

1986-1987   Distinguished Research Fellow, Mary E. Switzer Distinguished Research Fellowship, U.S. Department of Education. "Fellowship on the Financing of Medical Rehabilitation Services." Developed a book, a monograph, and an article on the financing and payment of Medical rehabilitation. $55,000. The publications are provided.

TEACHING

My general philosophy and approach to teaching are discussed at length in my personal statement. I believe that my teaching capabilities have improved every year at FIU, and I now feel that I am a strong classroom teacher. I am told that my students consider my courses rigorous. I am gratified that, despite this or hopefully because of it, my classes are popular, often requiring a change of venue to a larger classroom than originally scheduled. I am currently teaching two large classes of 85 and 45 students respectively.

I have enormous respect for my students, many of whom must drag themselves to my class at night after a hard day of work, child rearing, and other challenges. I am proud that most of them have reciprocated in treating me with similar respect and appreciation, as reflected in my student evaluations. All together, about 59% of my 643 student evaluations indicated that my overall teaching is excellent; about 88% found that I was either excellent or very good; and fully 98% concluded that I was excellent, very good or good. A summary table of my overall evaluations is provided below.

The following are the courses I have taught at FIU and the semesters in which I have taught them:

HSA #3103   Health and Social Service Systems
Summer 1999
Fall 1999
Spring 2000
Summer 2000
Fall 2000
Fall 2001
Spring 2002
Summer 2002
Fall 2002

HSA #4421   Legal Aspects and Legislation in Health Care

Summer 1998
Fall 1998
Spring 1999
Summer 1999
Fall 1999
Spring 2000
Summer 2000
Fall 2000
Spring 2001
Fall 2001
Spring 2002
Fall 2002

HSA #4150   People, Power and Politics

Summer 2002

PAD #4034   Policy Analysis and Program Evaluation

Spring 1998

HSA #5125   Introduction to Health Services

Fall 1998
Spring 1999
Summer 1999

HSA #6426   Health Law and Legal Aspects of Management

Fall 1997
Summer 1998
Summer 1999
Spring 2000
Spring 2001

Spring 2002

HSA #6155   Health Economics and Policy
Fall 1997
Spring1998
Summer 1998
Spring 1999
Summer 1999
Summer 2000

SERVICE

One of the things I enjoy most about being a member of the
FIU faculty is the opportunity to provide service to the
community. As I discuss in my personal statement, I have a
long-standing commitment to public service dating back to
my high school days. I believe that my service activities have
been extensive, and have been provided at every level from
local to national. The following are my service activities:

OFFICES HELD IN PROFESSIONAL ORGANIZATIONS

1989-pres.   *Journal of Disability Policy Studies*: Academic
              journal based at the University of Arkansas.
              (Sponsor of the Batavia Writing Competition
              on Disability Policy 1992-96.)
              1989-99: Founding Associate Editor.

2000-pres   Member, Editorial Board and Guest Editor.

1997-pres.   Board Member, Death with Dignity National
              Center: organization dedicated to improving

end-of-life care and enhancing options for people with terminal illnesses.

OTHER PROFESSIONAL ACTIVITIES AND PUBLIC SERVICE

Public Commission Membership (Appointments)

1997-pres.   Co-Chairperson, Barrier-Free Environment Committee, Miami Beach, Florida.

1998-pres.   Member (Ex-officio), Design Review Board, Miami Beach, Florida.

1999-2000   Commissioner, Occupational Access and Opportunity Commission (OAOC), recommended by Governor Bush and appointed by the Speaker of the House of the State of Florida.

1997-98   Board Member, Housing Finance Authority, Miami-Dade County, Florida (appointed by County Commissioner Bruce Kaplan).

1992-1993   Member, ADA Insurance Task Force, President's Committee on Employment of People With Disabilities.

1991-1992   Member, Long-Term Planning Advisory Group, National Institute on Disability and Rehabilitation Research.

1990-1992   Member, Insurance Advisory Committee, National Council on Disability.

1990-1991   Member, Task Force on Medical Rehabilitation Research, National Institutes of Health.

1975-1980   Member of Mayor's Committee for Housing of the Disabled, Riverside, California.

Board Membership (Private Sector)

2002-Pres.   Founding Chairman and President, AUTONOMY, Inc. Disability rights organization dedicated to furthering the self-determination of people with disabilities in all aspects of their lives. See www. Autonomy-now.org.

1988-1990   Editorial Board Member, *Assistive Technology*:
Academic journal based at the Department of Mechanical Engineering of the Massachusetts Institute of Technology (MIT).

1989-1990   Co-Founder and Board Member, Independent Living Assistance, Inc.:
Established with Louise McKnew and Robert McFarlane a non-profit corporation to research and develop demonstration projects to provide personal assistance and other independent living services to persons with disabilities.

1987-1990   Founding President and Chairman of Board of
             Directors, AIB Unlimited, Inc.:
             Established non-profit corporation to develop
             and market products designed or adapted to
             enhance the independence and personal
             satisfaction of persons who are physically
             disabled or elderly.

1988-1989   Vice President and Member of Board of
             Directors, Town Square Towers, Inc.:
             Elected to term on the five member Board of
             Directors of Town Square Towers, a
             condominium in Southwest Washington, DC,
             with 280 apartment units and an annual budget
             of over $1 million.

1982-1984   Founding President and Member of Board of
             Directors, Stanford Disabled Students:
             Established with several other graduate
             students at Stanford University a student
             organization for the purpose of representing
             the interests of students and others with
             disabilities on campus.

Other Committee Participation

2000   Member, Americans with Disabilities for
             Democracy.

1999-pres.   Member, Advisory Committee for *Disability
             Agenda*, National Organization on Disability,
             Washington DC.

1996-pres.	Advisory Board Member, Rehabilitation Research and Development Center on Managed Care and Disability (funded by NIDRR, U.S. Department of Education).
1999-2000	Member, Disability Advisory Committee, and Member, Health Care Advisory Committee, McCain 2000 presidential campaign.
1998	Jeb Bush for Governor Campaign, Miami-Dade County, Florida.
1997	Member, Downtown Transportation Committee, Greater Miami Chamber of Commerce.
1994-1995	Member, National Steering Committee on Managed Care for Persons and Persons with Disabilities, National Academy for State Health Policy.
1994-1995	Member, National Advisory Panel on the Future of Community-Based Long-term Care, National Academy of Aging.
1995	Deputy Chairperson, National Disability Coalition, Dole for President Campaign.
1992	Member, Conference Planning Steering Committee for the Participatory Action Research Development Conference, NIDRR.

1992   Judge, National Organization on Disability's
                "Calling on America" Campaign Competition.

1992   Member, Campaign Council of Senior
                Advisors, and Member, Executive Committee
                on Disability Issues, Bush-Quayle 1992
                Presidential Campaign.

1989-1991   Member, Advisory Committee for the Report
                to Congress on "Health Insurance Issues
                Affecting Individuals With Disabilities and
                Chronic Conditions," Berkeley Planning
                Associates.

1984-1986   Member, "Special Mergers and Acquisitions
                Review Team," Health Care Financing
                Administration: Responsibilities included
                providing legal counsel for Committee
                charged by Congress with responsibility to
                review hospital mergers for their Medicare
                reimbursement implications, and to provide
                policy guidance for the Medicare treatment of
                future hospital mergers.

1982-1983   Member, "President's Committee for Policy
                On The Disabled," Stanford University:
                Responsibilities included developing, drafting,
                and presenting the "Policy Statement on
                Disability at Stanford" to Donald Kennedy,
                President of Stanford University.

1975-1980   Member of Chancellor's Committee on the
                Disabled, UC Riverside.

University Service

2000-pres. Member, Faculty Advisory Committee for the new Law School, Florida International University.

1998-2000 Member, Steering Committee, School of Policy and Management, Florida International University.

1999-2000 Member, Search Committee, School of Policy and Management, Florida International University.

Congressional Testimony

Statement on the Lethal Drug Abuse Prevention Act of 1998, S. 2151, Before the Committee on the Judiciary, United States Senate, 105th Congress, July 31, 1998.

Statement on the Technology-Related Assistance for Individuals With Disabilities Act of 1988 Before the Subcommittee on Select Education, Committee on Education and Labor, House of Representatives, June 30, 1988.

Presented written testimony on reforming the Social Security disability programs, which was published in the Congressional Record.

Pro Bono Appellate & Supreme Court Experience

Co-Counsel with Cleary, Gottlieb in New York on the Brief Amici on Behalf of AUTONOMY, Inc. et al. in the case of *Oregon v. Ashcroft*, Oregon District Court, 2002, and in the current appeal to the Ninth Circuit Court of Appeals.

Attorney of Record/primary author of the Brief Amici on Behalf of the Gay Men's Health Crisis, LAMDA Legal Defense and Education Fund, and Five Prominent Americans with Disabilities in Support of Respondents in *Washington v. Glucksberg* and *Vacco v. Quill* before the U.S. Supreme Court (right to physician-assisted dying case), 1996.

Attorney of record/primary author of the Brief Amici on Behalf of a Coalition of Floridians and Other Americans with Disabilities in Support of Respondents in *Krischer v. McIver,* 1997.

Other Service Activities

1990-pres.   Manuscript peer reviewer for several journals, including *The New England Journal of Medicine*, *Health Affairs*, the *Archives of Physical Medicine and Rehabilitation*, and the *Journal of Disability Policy Studies*.

AFFILIATIONS AND MEMBERSHIPS

Member, Bar of the State of Florida, Admitted 1996.

Member, Bar of the U.S. Supreme Court, Admitted May 1991.

Adjunct faculty member, Department of Community and Family Medicine, Georgetown University School of Medicine, Appointed June 1988.

Member, Bar of the District of Columbia, Admitted August 1988.

Member, State Bar of California, Admitted December 1984.

Fellow, Washington Academy of Sciences, Elected December 1987.

Lifetime Member, Kennedy Institute of Ethics, Georgetown University, Admitted November 1988.

Lifetime Member, Stanford Alumni Association.

Lifetime Member, University of California, Riverside, Alumni Association.

AWARDS AND HONORS

I am deeply honored to have been recognized nationally for my work on several occasions and by a variety of organizations, including the White House, the U.S. Department of Education, and the University Of California. The Department of Education has recognized me twice as a distinguished researcher. My alma mater, the University of California at Riverside, gave me the honor of presenting the graduation address ten years after my own graduation and bestowed upon me the Chancellor's Award, which had previously been given to only a few individuals, including President Ford. My service to the State of Florida has also earned me positive recognition. The following are my various awards and honors:

Mary E. Switzer Distinguished Research Fellowship in Long-Term Care, Awarded by the National Institute on Disability and Rehabilitation Research (NIDRR), U.S. Department of Education, 2001.

Certificate of Appreciation, Occupational Access and Opportunity Commission, State of Florida.

Included in Marquis Who's Who in the World, Millennium Edition.

Included in Marquis Who's Who in America, 87th Edition.

Included in Marquis Who's Who in American Law—11th Edition, Millennium Edition (in press).

Chancellor's Award, University of California at Riverside, June 17, 1995.

Commencement Speaker, University of California at Riverside Graduation, June 17, 1995.

Admitted to the Bar of the United States Supreme Court at the recommendation of U.S. Attorney General Dick Thornburgh, 1991.

Certificate of Appreciation, U.S. Department of Justice, 1991.

White House Fellowship, 1990-91, awarded by the President's Commission on White House Fellowships, appointed by the President, June 4, 1990.

Washington Academy of Sciences Fellow, elected December 1, 1987.

Mary E. Switzer Distinguished Research Fellow in Medical Rehabilitation Finance, Awarded by the National Institute on Disability and Rehabilitation Research (NIDRR), U.S. Department of Education, September 1986.

National Federation of Insurance Counsel Writing Competition—Second Place, 1982.

Dr. Paul Mitchell Humanitarian Scholarship, "for promoting human welfare and social reform," 1975.